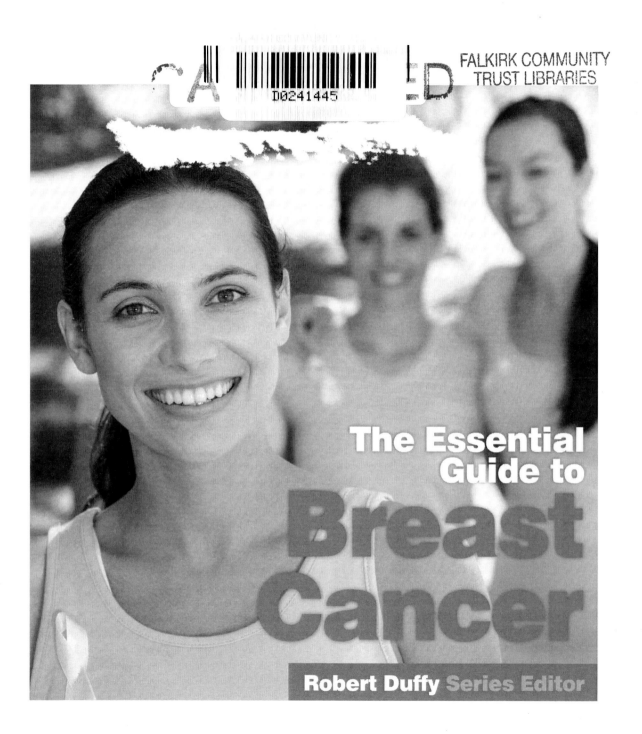

The Essential Guide to

Breast Cancer

Robert Duffy Series Editor

Published in Great Britain in 2017 by
need2know
Remus House
Coltsfoot Drive
Peterborough
PE2 9BF
Telephone 01733 898103
www.need2knowbooks.co.uk

Contents

Foreword

Being diagnosed with breast cancer is always a shock. It is a frightening and worrying time and events can happen quickly that make the situation seem quite overwhelming. The first instinct for most people is to try to find out as much as they can about the disease and the treatments on offer. Finding up-to-date, clear, accessible information can be difficult, and we always welcome any additional material that can help support women and their families during a time when people are often feeling lost and confused.

This book is written from the perspective of someone who has been through the experience of having breast cancer and has lived through the entire journey: from diagnosis, to treatment, to post-cancer care. As such, it offers an insider's guide to the most common concerns and questions. It also contains plenty of matter-of-fact advice on the practical and emotional implications at each stage of treatment.

It is our hope that having access to clear information will help women to feel empowered and that it will contribute towards them being well prepared to participate in any decisions that might be necessary throughout their journey.

Lorraine Sers and Anne Saunders

Macmillan breast nurse specialists

Introduction

This book has been written for anyone looking for straightforward information about breast cancer. The breast cancer journey can be a complex one – there are many different types of breast cancer and various treatments available, so your experience will be very much 'individual'. There is a lot of conflicting advice about the causes and treatment of cancer and I hope that the information in this book will give you a clear starting point to find your way through the maze of information available.

Often, an initial breast cancer diagnosis can leave everyone in shock. Many people will not have had any experience of serious illness before, and breast cancer affects the whole family, not just the person diagnosed. If you have been affected by breast cancer or have just received a diagnosis, hopefully this book will give you the plain advice needed to determine the best way forward for you and your family.

I was diagnosed with grade 2 lobular breast cancer in 2007. My initial reaction was to try to find out as much as possible about the disease and the treatments available. I was amazed at the amount of information out there – much of it conflicting. Although the Internet is a wonderful thing, and I have used it extensively in researching this book, the sheer amount of information can be overwhelming. It is my hope that this book has pared the plethora of information down to the bone and given anyone interested in breast cancer the best possible starting point.

There are many facts and figures about cancer in general and breast cancer in particular. The World Health Organisation have predicted that one in three people will be affected by some type of cancer during their lifetime and that the worldwide cancer rate will rise by 45% by 2030.

The World Health Organisation (WHO) is also doing a lot of work on raising awareness about cancer prevention. Their research shows that up to 30% of cancer cases could be prevented by modifying lifestyle or avoiding known risk factors. Risk factors for cancer generally include:

- Tobacco use.
- Being overweight or obese.

- Low fruit and vegetable intake.

- Physical inactivity.

- Alcohol use.

- A sexually transmitted HPV-infection (human papillomavirus).

- Urban air pollution.

- Indoor smoke from household use of solid fuels.

Breast cancer is now the most common cancer in the UK. In 2007, there were 45,700 women diagnosed with breast cancer. This figure equates to 125 new cases per day (Cancer Research UK, 2010). The incidence of breast cancer has increased by 50% in the last 25 years. Breast cancer has been likened to an epidemic, because there are so many new cases and the rates are increasing so rapidly.

On the plus side, survival rates for breast cancer are constantly and consistently on the rise. Almost two in three women with breast cancer now survive beyond 20 years from their initial diagnosis. There is new research coming through all the time and the outcomes for women with breast cancer are becoming more optimistic each year.

Disclaimer

This book is intended for general information only and is not intended to replace medical advice. You should always consult your GP for individual medical advice about breast cancer treatment. The factual material in this book is drawn from a variety of sources, which are listed at the back of this book. Please refer to those sources for the most up-to-date information.

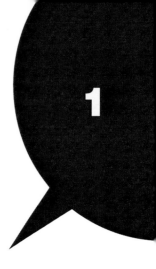

1

What is Breast Cancer?

Cancer

Cancer is best described as a disease in which abnormal (or malignant) cells divide and multiply without any order or control. These abnormal cells are unable to perform the functions they were designed for, for example to replace worn out cells or to repair damaged ones. The abnormal cells continue to grow and multiply without restraint; they do not respond appropriately to the body's signals to divide only when needed and to stop when that need is fulfilled. It is as though these cells have taken on a life of their own, ignoring the body's signals to maintain optimum health.

A tumour is formed when millions of these cells have divided and grown in one place (or site). The cancerous, or malignant, cells if left untreated will destroy healthy tissue and can spread and grow in other areas of the body, carried around in the bloodstream or lymphatic system.

'If we know what causes cells to become malignant, we can do more to prevent it occurring, but there is yet to be a definitive answer.'

The first question a person will ask when diagnosed with cancer is often 'Why does this happen?' or 'What causes abnormal cells?' – and scientists are working on these questions all the time. If we know what causes cells to become malignant, we can do more to prevent it occurring, but there is yet to be a definitive answer. We do know, however, that the DNA (genetic code) of these abnormal cells has somehow been damaged. Not all damaged cells go on to become cancer, but there are three primary reasons why damaged cells do become cancerous. These are:

- A mistake is made in the normal cell division process.
- Factors outside the body cause damage to the cells.
- Damaged DNA is inherited.

For the cells with damaged DNA to become cancerous, the body's own control system must fail. That means that the specific genes designed to look for damaged DNA and stop its production, do not do so.

When these malignant cells are found in the breast, the disease is called breast cancer. Even if the breast cancer cells divide and invade other areas of the body, it is still termed breast cancer because the invading cells are abnormal breast cells.

All cancers, including breast cancer, start with just one rogue cell. These single abnormal cells are usually found in the ducts or lobules of the breast. This is because these are the places where rapid cell division and growth occur naturally during the menstrual cycle.

There are two hormones that signal to the body to increase cell division and these are oestrogen and progesterone. Knowing which hormone is the trigger for normal and cancerous cells to grow and divide can help you understand some of the different types of treatment offered to you.

It can take months, or even years, before there is a mass of cells, or tumour, large enough to be detected by touch or a mammogram.

The breast

The breasts are mammary glands and their primary purpose is milk production. Each breast consists of 15 to 20 sections called lobes. Each lobe is made up of smaller sections called lobules, which are individual milk glands.

Within each lobe, there is a system of small tubes, or ducts, which carry the milk towards the nipples. The tissue surrounding the lobes consists mainly of fat (which is why breast shape can change when weight is lost or gained).

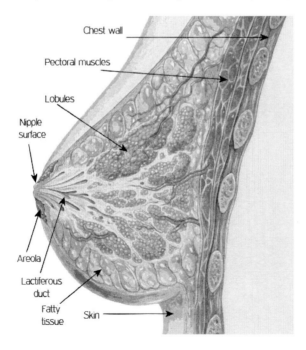

© Patrick J Lynch.

The breast is composed of:

- Milk glands (lobules which produce milk).
- Ducts that transport milk to the nipples.
- Areola (the pink or brown area around the nipple).
- Connective tissue which surrounds the lobules and ducts.
- Fat.

Case study

'When I was first diagnosed with breast cancer, I imagined a huge black monster inside me, eating away at my breast. I was absolutely terrified and spent the first week in tears. It was as though an alien had invaded my body. When I started to read a bit more about what cancer is, about how the damaged cells are not responding properly, it actually made me feel a lot better. I thought, if these cells can go wrong, surely they can be made right again? The more I knew, the more in control I felt. Instead of thinking that the disease was bigger than me, I started to feel that I was bigger than the disease.' Helen.

There are natural changes in shape that take place during the menstrual cycle. Breast shape changes most profoundly during pregnancy and breastfeeding, when the breasts are preparing or doing the job of delivering milk to the baby. It is not uncommon for a woman's breast size to go up one or two cup sizes during pregnancy. The most rapid change takes place in the first eight weeks.

The breasts change again during and after menopause. The breasts' glandular tissue, which has been kept firm so that the glands could produce milk, shrinks and is replaced with fatty tissue. The breasts also tend to increase in size and sag because the fibrous (connective) tissue loses its strength. Because the breasts become less dense after menopause, it is often easier for radiologists to detect breast cancer on an older woman's mammogram films, since abnormalities are not hidden by breast density.

Symptoms of breast cancer

Benign lumps

Very often, the first sign of breast cancer is a noticeable lump in the breast. However, 90% of breast lumps are benign (meaning they are not cancerous), but it is always worth having any lump checked by a GP. Most benign lumps are caused by natural changes in the body, particularly around the time of your period. Benign breast lumps do not turn into cancer.

There are many different types of benign breast lump, with various causes. These are:

- Areas of breast cell changes, more obvious around a period and more noticeable in over 35s.

- Cysts – sacs of fluid in the breast tissue are common, particularly in women before the menopause. Cysts can appear suddenly and it is not unusual to have several at the same time.

- Fibroadenoma – more common in younger women, these are collections of fibrous glandular tissue.

- Abscess or inflammation which is usually the result of an infection and treated with antibiotics.

- Lipoma – this is just a fatty lump.

- Periductal masitis – this is a rare condition, which is most commonly found in smokers. It is an inflammation and infection around the nipple area.

- Hamartoma – excessive growth that occurs in a small area of the breast.

- Fat necrosis – firm lumps that occur due to damage of fatty breast tissue, most usually from a bruise or injury.

- Papilloma – this growth is similar to a wart and develops inside a duct behind the nipple. These can be a naturally occurring symptom of getting older, but very rarely they are associated with another condition (atypical hyperplasia) that can develop into breast cancer.

- Fibrocystic disease or benign mammary change – caused by an overgrowth and thickening of fibrous tissue in an otherwise normal breast.

'Very often the first sign of breast cancer is a noticeable lump in the breast. However, 90% of breast lumps are benign.'

- Phyllodes tumours – these are lumps that can be either benign or malignant.

Although benign breast lumps can be annoying and worrying, they are usually harmless. There is no treatment for small fibroadenomas, hamartomas or lipomas unless they are causing symptoms.

Some other types of benign breast lump may require treatment. Cysts, for example, can be drained (aspirated) with a fine needle if they are very large. They don't usually require any further treatment.

Large fibroadenomas, hamartomas and lipomas are usually removed to prevent them getting larger still. They will be examined in a laboratory to be certain of the diagnosis.

Phyllodes lumps and papillomas are also always removed for diagnosis. It is worth remembering that these types of lumps are rare.

Case study

'I had always really liked my breasts! They were the only part of my body I felt confident about. They were always a good size and shape – not too big and not too small – and felt just right for me. I also very much enjoyed breastfeeding my two children. I fed Ollie for 12 months and William for eight. These were very special times and I really appreciated having the opportunity to bond with my babies in that way. I remember feeding alone at night and the sense of quiet and peace that filled the house.' Sarah.

Other breast symptoms

As well as the obvious lump in the breast, there are other breast changes that should be taken seriously and need to be checked by a GP.

Some changes which should be taken seriously are:

- A lump or thickening in an area of your breast.
- A change in the size or shape of your breast.
- Dimpling of the skin.
- A change in the shape of your nipple, particularly if it turns in, sinks into the breast or becomes irregular in shape.

- A blood-stained discharge from the nipple.

- A rash on your nipple or surrounding area.

- A swelling or lump in your armpit.

These symptoms do not necessarily mean cancer, they all can be attributed to other conditions, but it is always worth checking with a GP. The earlier breast cancer is detected, the more likely it is to be treated successfully. Very early breast cancers are easier to treat, may need less treatment and are more likely to be cured.

If your GP has any concerns about the lump, you will be sent to the breast clinic for further tests. This is what is called Triple Assessment and consists of clinical assessment (manual check), a mammogram and then possibly an ultrasound examination as the third stage.

At the breast clinic, a doctor will examine your breasts manually and ask about your medical history. The purpose of a mammogram, or ultrasound scan, is to establish the nature of the lump. A mammogram is a type of x-ray which can tell if the lump is solid (possible cancer) or filled with fluid (as in a benign cyst). Two radiologists will look at the results of your mammogram. If they are in any doubt about what they find, they will refer you for further testing. Many women will be familiar with an ultrasound scan from pregnancy. This type of scan uses sound waves to produce an image of the inside of your breast. Again, this is to establish the type of lump and appropriate treatment.

'The earlier breast cancer is detected, the more likely it is to be treated successfully. Very early breast cancers are easier to treat, may need less treatment and are more likely to be cured.'

Case study

'When I first referred to the breast clinic, I wasn't at all worried. I'd had my breasts checked eight months before and thought that I was just prone to lumpy breasts. However, when I got there it all became a bit scarier. I waited ages for the mammogram, but I was lucky that there was a radiologist on site who was able to look at the results immediately. She referred me for biopsy there and then. I wasn't really prepared for it and suddenly it seemed that everyone was taking this very seriously indeed. It felt as though I was rushed onto a conveyor belt of testing. I remember thinking "I've got to get home to make dinner for the kids", but they kept on and wouldn't let me go home. In retrospect, it was probably their fast reactions that saved my life.' Kate.

Depending on the results of your clinical assessment, mammogram and/or ultrasound, they will decide if you need a biopsy on the lump. A biopsy means taking a small sample of cells or tissue from the breast and examining it under a microscope. From this, doctors can tell if the lump is made up of cancerous cells. A biopsy is most often performed under local anaesthetic and is a relatively quick procedure.

NHS Breast Screening Programme

The NHS Breast Screening Programme for women over 50 has been running since 1988.

The programme provides free screening for women over 50 every three years. Around one and half million women take up the screening every year; however, not every woman will receive an invitation for screening immediately when she reaches 50, but all women should certainly have been screened by the age of 53. This is because each health authority operates a rolling programme, so if you have just missed a screening session when you turn 50, you will have to wait another three years for the programme to roll around again.

The programme doesn't include women under the age of 50 for two main reasons. Firstly, the incidence of breast cancer is much lower in this age range. Secondly, breast cancer is much harder to detect in pre-menopausal women, as the density of the breast tissue is different. There are some moves to extend the breast screening programme to include women from 47 and up to the age of 73 (currently the cut off age is 70). After the age of 70 you can still request breast screenings and they will still be free, but you will no longer be part of the programme and won't receive automatic appointments.

Breast screening involves taking an x-ray of each breast. This is called a mammogram and it involves placing the breast between two metal plates in order for the image to be taken. Most women find it mildly uncomfortable, but it only lasts for a very short time – probably around 30 seconds per breast. The x-ray is capable of detecting small changes that would not be felt by self-examination or by examination from a doctor.

The appointment itself takes around half an hour. A receptionist, or mammogram operator, will take your personal details, such as name, age and address. The mammogram operator will then ask you a little about your medical history; for example, they may ask if you have any history of breast lumps and if you have noticed any symptoms that you are concerned about.

The results of your mammogram will be sent to your GP within about two weeks. A percentage will be recalled for further tests or another mammogram. A certain proportion of these will be because the results were unclear because of technical difficulties with the x-ray.

In between screenings, or for those women who are under 50 and not yet part of the NHS Breast Screening Programme, the Department of Health recommend being breast aware. There is no evidence to show that a formal self-examination technique performed every month at around the same time lowers the fatality rate for breast cancer. Instead, the Department of Health recommend a more relaxed approach and to be aware of what is normal (or not) for you. Every woman is different and the size, shape and feel of breasts will vary enormously from person to person. You can download a leaflet with more information about being breast aware from the NHS at www.cancerscreening.nhs.uk.

There has been some negative publicity recently about what has been termed as 'over screening'. This is where small anomalies in the breast are picked up and treatment commences, when it might prove not to be necessary. However, research conducted by Stephen Duffy (2010) shows that the benefits of screening clearly outweigh the perceived harm of over diagnosis. The study suggests that between two and two-and-a-half lives are saved for every over diagnosed case.

The evidence for breast screening is overwhelmingly positive. The World Health Organisation International Agency for Research on Cancer (IRAC) (2002) collected evidence from 11 participating countries and concluded that there is a 35% reduction in fatalities from breast cancer in those countries that implement a breast screening programme. This translates into one saved life for every 500 women screened.

If you miss your breast screening appointment then you are free to rearrange it at any time by getting in touch with the local screening unit. If you don't rearrange the appointment, you will be invited again as part of the next three yearly cycle, but you are free to rearrange the appointment at any point until you are invited again. Contact details for local units are available in the Yellow Pages or on the NHS website through the postcode finder.

Summing Up

- Cancer occurs when cells divide and multiply out of control. A tumour is formed when millions of cells have divided and grown in one site.

- 90% of breast lumps are benign (non-cancerous), but you should always get anything unusual checked by your GP.

- The earlier breast cancer is detected, the more likely it will be treated successfully.

- Women over 50 will be offered a mammogram every three years as part of the NHS Breast Screening Programme.

- Regular breast screening for women over 50 is proven to reduce breast cancer related fatalities by 35%.

- A relaxed approach to breast awareness is as effective as formal self-examination.

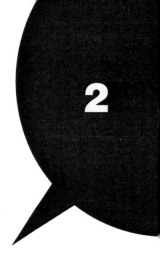

2

Causes and Risks of Breast Cancer

The risks of developing breast cancer fall into three categories. They are:

- Definite risks.
- Hormonal risks.
- Lifestyle and medical history risks.

Definite risks

Definite risks include:

- Getting older.
- Carrying the breast cancer gene.
- Having had breast cancer before.

Getting older

Getting older increases the risk of any disease. The older the person, the higher the chances of cells in the body producing cancer cells, simply because there is more time for it to happen. This is why free mammograms are offered to women between the ages of 50 to 70 as part of the screening programme in the UK.

Breast cancer in the family

Breast cancer in the family can sometimes increase the chances of developing breast cancer. Compared to the general population, your risk may be increased if you have one of the following in your family history:

- A mother or sister diagnosed with breast cancer before the age of 40.
- Two close relatives from the same side of the family diagnosed with breast cancer – at least one must be a mother, sister or daughter.
- Three close relatives diagnosed with breast cancer at any age.
- A father or brother diagnosed with breast cancer at any age.
- A mother or sister with breast cancer in both breasts – the first cancer diagnosed before the age of 50.
- One close relative with ovarian cancer and one with breast cancer, diagnosed at any age – at least one must be a mother, sister or daughter.

(Source: CancerHelp UK, 2010).

The affected members of your family must be blood relatives (that is, either from your mother's or father's side of the family). If your risk is high, you may be offered an appointment with a genetic counsellor to determine your risk and suggest steps to minimise it.

Carrying the breast cancer gene

Breast cancer genes are hard to identify. There are probably several genes that increase the risk of breast cancer, and currently it is possible to test for two of them. They are BRCA 1 and BRCA 2. Carrying these genes means that you have a higher than average risk of getting breast cancer, but it does not mean you will definitely get breast cancer. The risk of developing cancer if you carry either of these genes could be up to 85%, but it is impossible to be more precise because actual risk will vary from family to family and between individuals.

There is another gene fault that can be tested called the TP53 Gene. This is much rarer than the BRCA mutations.

Having had breast cancer before

Having had breast cancer before increases your risk of getting it in the other breast. This is why you are called back for regular mammograms and check ups in the early years after a breast cancer diagnosis (usually up to five years). It means that any cancer will be picked up and treated quickly. Some cancer treatment drugs, such as Tamoxifen, can reduce the risk of developing cancer in the other breast.

Hormonal risks

Sex hormones

We all have male and female hormones in our bodies and the risk of breast cancer seems to be affected by both. Oestrogen and progesterone have always been cited as risk factors in developing breast cancer, but now it has been confirmed by studies conducted by EPIC (European Prospective Investigation of Cancer) that high levels of testosterone can raise a women's risk of pre-menopausal and possibly post-menopausal breast cancer.

Periods starting very early or finishing late can increase the risk of breast cancer. The early onset of menarche (starting periods) is linked to a higher risk. Similarly, a late menopause can increase the risk of developing breast cancer. Early means around the age of 11 and a late menopause means after the age of 54. It is unclear why these factors might increase risk, but one theory is that the body is exposed to the hormone oestrogen for longer.

Children

The age at which a woman has children also appears to affect the risk of developing breast cancer. Women who have never had children are at slightly increased risk, as are women who have their first baby after the age of 35. Generally, the younger a woman is when she has her first baby, the lower the risk of developing breast cancer. However, having children very young has been shown to slightly increase the risk of cervical cancer.

'Some studies suggest that a healthy, balanced diet could prevent up to 15% to 35% of cancers.'

Hormone replacement therapy

Hormone replacement therapy (HRT) comes in two varieties. One contains just oestrogen and the other has both oestrogen and progesterone in a single pill. It is the HRT treatment containing both hormones that appears to dramatically increase breast cancer risk, although long-term use of the oestrogen-only pill (over 20 years) also appears to increase risk.

In 2003, Cancer Research UK looked specifically at HRT and breast cancer risks, which proved for the first time that there was an increased risk of developing breast cancer while taking HRT.

Taking HRT has to be a personal decision taken on an individual basis with the advice of a medical professional.

The contraceptive pill

The effect of taking the contraceptive pill on the increased risk of breast cancer is unclear at the moment. The pill contains oestrogen, which can stimulate breast cancer cells to grow. Some studies show a slight increased risk of developing cancer while taking the pill, while others show no increased risk. There is a need for more research in this area.

It is also worth remembering that breast cancer is less usual in younger women, who are more likely to be taking the pill.

Lifestyle risks

Diet

More research is being undertaken on the effect of diet on all cancers (not just breast cancer). Some studies suggest that a healthy, balanced diet could prevent up to 15% to 35% of cancers.

One way of being able to prove this is by looking at breast cancer rates and diets from around the world. The most common example being the very low rate of breast cancer amongst Japanese women, who traditionally have a diet low in saturated fat and high in vegetables and soy products.

However, it is very difficult to draw firm conclusions about diet and cancers because of variations in diet over a person's lifetime. There is currently a major study being undertaken by European Prospective Investigation into Cancer (EPIC), started in 1992, which is following people's eating habits over a set period of time and then following up to see which illnesses develop in later life.

It is proven, however, that a diet high in fresh fruit and vegetables and low in saturated fats and sugars is best for preventing cancer as well as other diseases, such as diabetes and heart disease.

So what is a healthy, balanced diet? Decreasing animal fats and processed sugar and replacing with a higher proportion of fresh fruit and vegetables is a very good start.

Current dietary advice includes:

- Replacing animal fats with polyunsaturated fats (found in some vegetable oils) and monounsaturated fats (such as those found in olive oil).

- Eating more fibre, found in wholegrains (such as oats, wheat and cereals), beans, fruits and vegetables.

- Eating more isoflavones, found primarily in soy, peas and beans and ligans (found in vegetables, fruits, wholegrains, tea and coffee).

- Keeping calcium levels up by eating dairy foods in moderation. Calcium is also found in green leafy vegetables such as broccoli or cabbage, but not in spinach. Soya beans, nuts, fish (such as sardines and pilchards), tofu and bread also contain calcium.

- Eating foods high in carotenoids – that is food that contains chemicals that the body changes into vitamin A. These include carrots, sweet potatoes, spinach and tomatoes.

For more information on healthy eating, see *Food for Health – The Essential Guide* (Need2Know).

Alcohol

Drinking alcohol slightly increases your risk of breast cancer. According to some studies (Zang *et al*, 2007), women who have three or four drinks a day increase their risk by about a third (33%).

There have been a lot of studies into alcohol consumption and breast cancer risk. Broadly, the findings show that out of 100 women, by the age of 80, the number who will develop breast cancer will be:

'Drinking alcohol slightly increases your risk of breast cancer. Women who have three or four drinks a day increase their risk by about a third (33%).'

- 8.8% if they don't drink at all.
- 10.1% if they have two drinks per day.
- 13.3% if they have six drinks per day.

(Source: Cancer Research UK, 2009).

There are two aspects of this research that are of interest. Firstly, the increased risk does not vary according to age, race, weight, family history or any of the other known risk factors.

Secondly, the research proves that the risk increases directly according to the number of drinks per day. For each additional drink, the risk increases by 7%.

Drinking alcohol is a small risk compared with other risk factors, but it is worth keeping within government guidelines of 14 units per week for women. A unit is the equivalent of a small glass of wine.

Weight

Being overweight after reaching the menopause increases the risk of breast cancer. Nine out of 100 women of a healthy weight will develop breast cancer by the age of 50, whereas 12 out of 100 overweight women will develop breast cancer by the age of 50 (Breakthrough Breast Cancer, 2006).

Strangely, being overweight before the menopause slightly decreases the risk of developing breast cancer. This may be because overweight women tend to ovulate less and therefore have less exposure to oestrogen. There are, of course, many other disease risks that are associated with being overweight at any age and maintaining a healthy body mass index (BMI) is crucial for a healthy lifestyle.

Body mass index chart

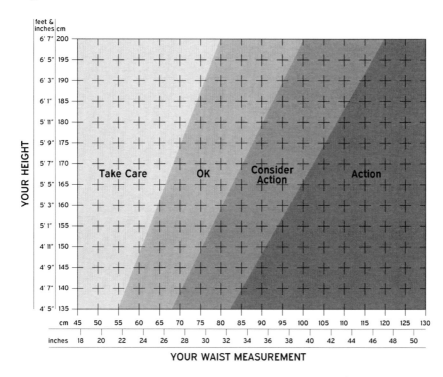

© Crown copyright. Source: Food Standards Agency.

'Exercise is known to help reduce the risk of developing breast cancer. Regular physical activity also lowers the risk of developing other diseases such as osteoporosis, heart disease and strokes.'

Exercise

Exercise is known to help reduce the risk of developing breast cancer. Regular physical activity also lowers the risk of developing other diseases such as osteoporosis, heart disease and strokes.

The government recommended amount of exercise is at least 30 minutes of moderate exercise five times per week. The type of exercise doesn't appear to make much difference; the important factors are amount and regularity.

Having an active lifestyle includes things like gardening, walking and vigorous housework. It doesn't always have to be going to the gym!

Smoking

Up until recently, researchers were divided as to whether smoking increased the risk of developing breast cancer. Although smoking is definitely linked to the dramatically increased risk of other types of cancer, such as lung or mouth, the link to breast cancer was less obvious.

'Breastfeeding does appear to lower the risk of developing breast cancer. The longer a woman breastfeeds, the lower the risk becomes.'

However, scientists now believe that smoking does carry an increased risk of developing breast cancer. One study showed that risk increase could be as high as 30% (Reynolds *et al.*, 2004). Although other studies show a much lower risk increase for breast cancer in smokers, the overall evidence is clear about the negative effect of smoking on general health.

Breastfeeding

Breastfeeding does appear to lower the risk of developing breast cancer. The longer a woman breastfeeds, the lower the risk becomes (Furberg *et al.,* 1999). The risk lowers by 4.3% for every year of breastfeeding and by 7% for each child born.

It is worth noting that 90% of Japanese women (where breast cancer rates are the lowest in the world) breastfeed.

Summing Up

- The risks of cancer occurring are diverse, some of which we have no control over and some of which we do.

- Definite risks, of which we have no control over, include: getting older, having breast cancer in the family, carrying the breast cancer gene and having had breast cancer before.

- Hormonal risks increase post-menopause as oestrogen and testosterone are present in high levels in our bodies. Taking HRT has also been implicated in an increased risk of developing breast cancer.

- A healthy, balanced diet is thought to have preventative effects on the risk of developing breast cancer. Cutting down on red meat and dairy products and increasing your fruit and vegetable intake are ways to improve your diet.

- Cutting down on alcohol, giving up smoking and maintaining a healthy weight are also important factors in leading a healthy lifestyle.

- The most important thing you can do is exercise. Keeping your body and organs in good shape should be a priority.

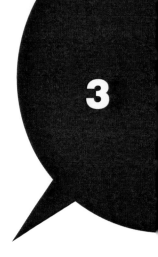

3

Tests and Diagnosis

Tests and diagnosis

Your GP

If there are any concerns about the possibility of having breast cancer, the first appointment will be a visit to your GP. Usually, your GP will examine you visually and manually. GPs do not have any specialist equipment for detecting breast cancer, so if they see anything even slightly unusual, they will make a quick referral to the breast clinic. Being referred to the breast clinic does not mean that you have cancer, it just means that further tests need to be taken.

The breast clinic

'Being referred to the breast clinic does not mean that you have cancer, it just means that further tests need to be taken.'

At the breast clinic the initial examination will almost always be manual. That is, a doctor will feel your breasts in order to gauge the extent of any unusual lumps. They will also look at the shape of your breasts and compare the size and shape of the two. This is to check if there are any visual differences. Checks will also be made to your neck and under the armpits to see if there are any lumps in the lymph gland system.

Ultrasound scan

If there is any doubt about the nature of the lump, the next step could be an ultrasound scan. An ultrasound scan uses sound waves to make a picture of the inside of the body. Younger women (under 35) are more likely to be offered an ultrasound scan. If a lump is detected, doctors will want to know what type it is. That is, if it is benign (non-cancerous) or malignant (cancerous). Ultrasound scans are not painful. An operator will put gel on your skin and move a microphone over the area in order to build a picture of the lump, exactly as an ultrasound during pregnancy.

Mammogram

A mammogram is an x-ray that can detect lumps in the breast that may be difficult to feel. If the results of the mammogram are unclear, you may be offered an ultrasound as well. Mammograms are offered as part of the breast screening programme in the UK to women between 50 and 70 years old every three years.

Mammograms can be slightly uncomfortable because the breast has to be placed between two metal plates in order for the x-ray to be taken. The plates close down on the breast, applying a little pressure for a minute or two. Although this can be uncomfortable, it is over very quickly.

After the mammogram, two radiologists will look at the x-rays and decide on the next step. Not all cancers show up on mammograms, so it is important to keep checking your breasts, even if you are having regular mammograms.

Biopsy

The third and more definitive tool used to detect cancer is a biopsy. Biopsy means taking a sample of tissue from the lump in the breast in order to check it for cancerous cells. There are several types of biopsy available.

The most usual biopsy performed in the breast clinic is a needle core biopsy. This is when a fine needle is used to extract a sample from the breast lump, which is then sent to the lab for testing. A needle core biopsy uses a local anaesthetic directly on the site of the lump. It only takes a minute or two and although it is not usually painful, it can be uncomfortable.

It is not always possible to get a good enough sample using this method and if that is the case, the next step is a needle biopsy performed under local anaesthetic. A needle biopsy uses a slightly larger needle in order to gather a larger sample for the lab. The samples from this type of test can tell the laboratory more about the type of cancer, as some tissue from the breast around the lump is also removed.

An incisional biopsy removes a portion of the lump. This is usually used for larger lumps and the procedure is done with a local anaesthetic. Usually, you will be sent home the same day.

There may be occasions when an excision biopsy is used. This requires a minor operation in hospital, in order for surgeons to remove the whole lump for testing. An excisional biopsy is usually performed in the outpatient department of your local hospital. Local anaesthetic is used and the procedure usually will take less than an hour. After a couple of hours' recovery time, you will usually be sent home that same day. You may experience some bruising, but any scar will be very small indeed.

Waiting for test results

Waiting for test results can be a very anxious time. How long you have to wait will vary depending on where you live. Some health authorities are able to issue results on the same day, while others may have a wait of up to two weeks.

Ask at the clinic how long the results will take. This may be a time when you need to talk to other people about their experiences and have the opportunity to express how you are feeling. The breast care nurses will be able to put you in touch with support groups in your local area if you ask them.

'Often, people find talking to others a great help, and finding the right sort of support can be very beneficial. It could be a formal group, or particular friends or family members.'

A breast cancer diagnosis

A cancer diagnosis can be very frightening. Many people describe it as the most traumatic event in their lives and it is very normal to be in a state of shock immediately afterwards. However, treatment for cancer is improving all the time and survival rates are now higher than ever.

Often, people find talking to others a great help, and finding the right sort of support can be very beneficial. It could be a formal group, or particular friends or family members. Sharing concerns with others can often help to put things in perspective and dispel any worries you may have.

A cancer diagnosis can raise many questions and there is so much information available that it can become confusing. Getting clear answers is the best way of understanding your particular type of cancer and the treatment options for it.

Questions to ask your doctor

Hospitals are busy places and it is easy to forget any questions you may have. It is a good idea to write questions down beforehand so that you are prepared when you see your specialist. It is also helpful to have someone else with you, and maybe that person can take notes. There may be a lot of information that is difficult to take in at one time.

Here is an example list of questions you may want to ask your doctor after a diagnosis of breast cancer.

- What type of breast cancer do I have?
- What is the stage and grade of my cancer?

- What are the outcomes for this type of cancer?
- What treatment do you recommend? Why is it best for me?
- What are the benefits of this treatment?
- What are the risks of this treatment?
- What are the side effects of this treatment?
- How successful is this treatment for my type of breast cancer?
- What will my life be like after treatment?
- What would happen if I decided against further treatment?
- Would you recommend a second opinion?
- I need time to think about things. Will it make a difference?

Sometimes people want to know what has caused the cancer; for example, does stress cause cancer? Is there something I have done to cause my cancer? Doctors find it very difficult to answer these questions, as no one really knows the answers. It may be more helpful to focus on getting well rather than on why the cancer has developed.

'Hospitals are busy places and it is easy to forget any questions you may have. It is a good idea to write questions down beforehand so that you are prepared when you see your specialist.'

Types of breast cancer

There are several different types of breast cancer, each with its own unique set of risks and possible treatments. The type of cancer you are diagnosed with will greatly affect your experience and journey.

Ductal carcinoma in situ

Ductal carcinoma in situ (DCIS) is the most common non-invasive cancer. DCIS occurs within the breast ducts and means the cancer has not yet spread to other areas of the breast or other parts of the body.

Invasive ductal breast cancer

Invasive ductal breast cancer is the most common type of breast cancer. Of all breast cancer diagnoses, 70-80% are this type of cancer. It is also sometimes referred to as ductal carcinoma as it describes a cancer that is growing in ducts in the breasts.

It is important to understand the difference between invasive and non-invasive cancers. If you have DCIS, you do not have invasive ductal cancer.

Lobular carcinoma in situ

Lobular carcinoma in situ (LCIS) is when changes occur in the cells inside the breast lobes. This is not strictly cancer, but does increase the risk of cancer developing. If you are diagnosed with LCIS, you will be monitored closely in case of cancer developing.

Invasive lobular breast cancer

Invasive lobular breast cancer accounts for approximately 10% of breast cancers. It means that the cancer has originated in the lobules of the breast. This type of breast cancer is most common in women between 45 and 55 years old.

Invasive lobular breast cancer can be difficult to diagnose, as it does not always show up as a lump. Because of this, it is also difficult to pick up with a mammogram. One physical symptom of invasive lobular breast cancer is a thickening area of the breast. This is another reason why it is important to be aware of how your breasts feel, so you are able to detect any changes.

Inflammatory breast cancer

Inflammatory breast cancer is a rare type of breast cancer. Only about 1 or 2% of all breast cancers are inflammatory. This type of cancer blocks the small lymph channels in the breast (the channels that drain away excess fluid from tissues and organs). Because of this blockage, the breast becomes inflamed; that is, swollen, hot, red and firm to the touch. It can occur quite suddenly and, as such, is easily confused with mastitis (an infection of the breast).

Treatment for inflammatory breast cancer can differ from other types of breast cancer. Often chemotherapy is offered first, before surgery, with radiotherapy or hormonal treatments being offered after surgery.

Paget's disease

Paget's disease is also an unusual type of breast cancer, occurring in only 1-2% of all new cases. This cancer starts in the nipple or the areola (dark area around the nipple). The first signs can be a red, scaly itchy rash, which can be mistaken for eczema. A biopsy will be taken, as very often there is a lump behind the nipple.

Rare types of breast cancer

Rare types of breast cancer affect less than 5% of cancers diagnosed. These are often referred to as 'special type', whereas the most common form of cancer (invasive ductal breast cancer) is referred to as 'no special type' and can be written in notes as 'NST' (no special type) or 'NOS' (not otherwise specified). Invasive lobular breast cancer is also referred to as a 'special type'.

Rare types of breast cancer include:

- Medullay breast cancer.
- Mucinous (or colloid) breast cancer.
- Tubular breast cancer.
- Adenoid cystic carcinoma.
- Papillary breast cancer.
- Metaplastic breast cancer.
- Angiosarcoma of the breast.
- Phyllodes or cytosarcoma phyllodes.
- Lymphoma of the breast.
- Basal type breast cancer.

Just because a cancer is rare does it mean that it's more difficult to treat. In fact, certain types of rare breast cancer (medullay, for example) can have better outcomes than more usual breast cancers. Most treatments for rare breast cancers are similar to those for usual types of breast cancer.

You can find out more about rare types of breast cancer from Cancer Help UK (see help list).

Breast cancer in men

Breast cancer in men is very rare. There are less than 300 cases every year in this country (compared with 45,000 women). Symptoms, diagnosis and treatments are very similar to breast cancer in women.

Often, men with a breast cancer diagnosis can feel very isolated – and if this is the case, it is important to get appropriate support. Some of the larger cancer charities have male volunteers who will be experienced in dealing with men with breast cancer, and Macmillan has a section on their website especially for men. Sadly, however, support can be lacking for male cancer sufferers.

Staging and grading of breast cancer

Stage and grade refer to two different things:

- Stage refers to the size of the cancer and whether it has spread beyond the original site.

- Grade refers to the extent of the cancer and how quickly it is likely to grow.

The number staging and grading system

The number staging system goes from 0-4. DCIS is often referred to as stage 0. This is because DCIS is almost always completely curable with treatment. Staging always refers to invasive breast cancer.

- Stage 1 – used to describe a cancer where the tumour is less that 2cm (1in) in diameter and there is no sign of any spread in other parts of the body.

- Stage 2 – when the tumour measures between 2-5cm (1-2in), or the lymph glands in the armpit are affected, or both together. Stage 2 shows no signs that the cancer has spread further.

- Stage 3 – when the tumour is larger than 5cm (2in) and may be attached to muscle or skin that surrounds it. Usually, the lymph nodes are also affected but there is no sign that the cancer has spread beyond the breast or lymph glands.

- Stage 4 – denotes a tumour of any size and there is evidence that the cancer has spread to other parts of the body. The lymph nodes are almost always affected. This is known as secondary or metastatic breast cancer. Breast cancer that comes back after initial diagnosis and treatment is called recurrent breast cancer.

Grading gives an idea of how quickly the cancer might develop (or grow). The grades range from 1-3.

- Grade 1 – low grade and means that the cancer cells look similar to the healthy cells in the breast.

- Grade 2 – an intermediate or moderate grade which falls between the two other grades. The level of activity for grade 2 cancers is likely to be between the other two.

- Grade 3 – high grade and denotes that the cancer cells look very abnormal under a microscope. These high-grade tumours are likely to grow quickly and are prone to spreading to other areas of the body.

For further information on staging and grading, please go to www.macmillan.org.uk.

Summing Up

- If there is a possibility that you may have breast cancer, there are several tests that can be done to determine a diagnosis. Waiting for test results will understandably be a stressful time. Ask your clinic when you should expect to receive the results as it will depend on where you live.

- Should you be diagnosed with breast cancer, you will inevitably have a lot of questions. Make notes during your consultations, or take along a loved one who can do this for you.

- There is a lot to think about immediately after a breast cancer diagnosis. You may find you have a million questions running through your head or really need to talk about it with other people who have been there. You may find the opposite is true and you need some time to get used to the idea before 'going public'.

- There are several different types of breast cancer, so your experience will very much depend on your diagnosis.

- The stage of cancer refers to the size and how far it has spread. The grade of cancer refers to the extent and how quickly it is likely to grow.

- It is important to take everything at your own pace and remember that it is entirely up to you how much or how little you want to talk about your cancer. This is your body and your life.

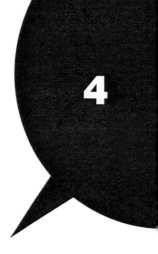

4

Breast Cancer Treatment

reast cancer treatments broadly consist of surgery, chemotherapy, radiotherapy and hormone therapy. The type of treatment you are offered will depend on the type of cancer you have, the stage and grade of your cancer, and also your age.

Surgery

Surgery to remove cancer still plays a fundamental role in cancer treatment. Surgery, which is an operation to repair or remove a malfunctioning body part, is used for a variety of reasons. Doctors use it to treat, or remove, the cancer, for accurate diagnosis or for relieving symptoms. Some patients will have surgery alone, while others will have surgery combined with other treatments. Many cancer patients will have all the treatment options available.

The primary purpose of cancer surgery is to remove the cancer from the body. The surgeon usually does this by removing the cancer and also a small amount of healthy tissue to ensure all of the cancer is removed. There are several types of surgery for breast cancer.

'The type of treatment you are offered will depend on the type of cancer you have, the stage and grade of your cancer, and also your age.'

Lumpectomy

A lumpectomy removes the lump from your breast and will take a little of the surrounding tissue for analysis. It is sometimes referred to as breast conserving surgery as only the lump is removed, not the whole breast. A lumpectomy is suitable for women who have only one lump, or only a small lump. It is not suitable if the cancer has spread, the lump is in a difficult position (for example, behind the nipple) or if the lump is particularly large.

Sometimes, radiotherapy or chemotherapy is offered before surgery. This is to shrink the lump and make surgery easier.

A lumpectomy is performed under a general anaesthetic, meaning you will be entirely asleep during the operation. As with all general anaesthetics, you will be required to fast for the morning before the operation. The operation usually takes around an hour and the incision will be stitched to close. This means you will have a dressing at the site of the operation and may want to wear a very light, soft bra afterwards.

Usually, you will stay in hospital for one night. It's important to rest until the effects of the anaesthetic have worn off and you will be required to have someone to take you home – driving after an anaesthetic is not recommended. You are usually advised not to drive, operate heavy machinery or make irreversible legal decisions (such as signing documents) for at least 48 hours after a general anaesthetic.

It can take up to a week to recover from a lumpectomy, so you may have to arrange to have time off work until you feel a bit better.

Axillary clearance

Lymph nodes perform the function of fighting infection, draining away fluids, waste products and damaged cells. They are mainly sited in the armpit, neck and groin areas. The axillary clearance only removes lymph nodes from under the armpit, where there can be up to 20 lymph nodes situated.

If the breast cancer has spread, it will go via the lymph nodes (also known as lymph glands) first before spreading to the rest of the body. Removing some or all of the lymph nodes in the armpit will ascertain whether the cancer has started to spread. However, even if cancer is detected in the lymph nodes, it does not necessarily mean that there is cancer in another part of your body.

Full removal of the lymph nodes is called an axillary clearance, but these days it is preferred to use minimal surgery rather than a full clearance.

Minimal surgery means performing sentinel lymph node biopsy (SLNB). This is the removal of the main (sentinel) lymph node only if abnormal lymph nodes are identified through ultrasound testing or ultrasound guided needle testing (during the ultrasound scan, the image is used to guide the needle towards the suspicious area in the breast).

SLNB is performed by using the duel technique of isotope and blue dye. The operation aims to remove the lymph node in the armpit where a breast cancer cell may first arrive. It is then looked at under the microscope. If there are no cancer cells seen at this site, it is unlikely that there will be any involvement in the remaining lymph nodes in the armpit. This operation has the advantage of being a smaller operation with fewer side effects than an operation to remove all the lymph nodes in your armpit.

The procedure involves an injection, during your operation, of a blue coloured dye which then enters the breast lymphatic vessels. The dye flows to the armpit and will usually colour the first lymph node, the sentinel node, blue. This is seen by your surgeon and removed. Occasionally, the sentinel node cannot be identified. In this situation, your surgeon will remove a few lymph nodes from the lower part of your armpit.

After your operation, you may wake up either in the recovery room adjoining the operating theatre or back on the ward. The nurses will monitor your pulse, blood pressure and wound to ensure you are recovering safely. It is usual to have an intravenous infusion (drip) in your arm to replace the fluid you lose during the operation. This will be removed once you are able to drink normally, usually later on your operation day.

You may have a drain in the wound. This is a small tube held by a stitch which drains into a plastic bag or bottle. It will be removed when the drainage has reduced, usually the day after your operation. You will have a scar where the sentinel node has been removed. It is joined with invisible stitches which gradually dissolve and will be covered with a dressing.

In order to help yourself in your recovery, it is important to do the following:

- Request painkillers or anti-sickness medication if you need them.

- Move your legs, feet and toes while you are in bed to help your blood flow. Get up and move around as soon as you feel safe and comfortable to do so. (It is important that a nurse is with you the first time that you get out of bed.)

The drains could be removed as early as the day after your operation, or it might be up to five days. Most women are sent home with the drain in place and it will then be removed by the district nursing team.

Some women report numbness in the area after an axillary operation and this is because some nerves will have been severed in order to remove the lymph nodes. Nerves do repair themselves and the majority of feeling should return within 12-18 months, although you may also experience stiffness in the arm and some pain and swelling in the area. It is recommended that you do not drive until you are confident that you could perform an emergency stop.

One possible side effect of having one or all the lymph nodes removed can be a build up of fluid in the affected arm. This is called lymphoedema and can be relieved with massage, but it is rarely completely cured. This will usually consist of gentle arm exercises, combined with massage to keep the area drained of fluid.

Women who have had lymph node surgery have to be careful about infection on that side of their body. Small cuts must be cleaned and covered, as the body will be less efficient at fighting infection on that side after the lymph nodes have been removed.

Mastectomy

A mastectomy is an operation that removes the whole breast. It is a larger operation than a lumpectomy, but the recovery rate is very good. There are two types of mastectomy – a simple mastectomy and a radical mastectomy. A simple mastectomy is when the breast tissue is removed. A radical mastectomy is when the breast tissue and underlying muscle from the chest wall is removed. A radical mastectomy is only required when the cancer has spread to the chest wall, and it is a much rarer operation.

A mastectomy is performed under a general anaesthetic and usually requires a hospital stay of at least one or two days, but it could be up to five days. The operation itself will take up to two hours.

After a mastectomy you will have some tubes (or drains) coming from the operation site, and you will also probably have a drip in your arm. Both of these are usually removed within two to three days. As the effects of the anaesthetic wear off, you will be offered pain-killers. The type of pain-killer you are offered will depend on the nature and severity of the discomfort.

Many hospitals will offer you a combination of exercises in order to restore strength and movement in your arm. The ward nurses and breast care team will show you how to perform these exercises.

If you haven't had an immediate breast reconstruction, you will be given a lightweight, foam bra insert called a Softie or a Comfie. This is worn for approximately six weeks, or until the scar has completely healed. Usually dissolvable stitches are used, which will disappear after about 10 days. Non-dissolvable stitches will be removed at a follow-up appointment a week or two after discharge from hospital.

You will then be offered an appointment to fit you with a suitable prosthesis, or false breast. These come in a variety of shapes and sizes and a trained fitter will be able to advise you on the best shape and size for you. They will match the shape of your existing breast as closely as possible. Breast prostheses are usually made of soft silicon and when worn under clothes can be indistinguishable from a natural breast.

Recovering from a mastectomy requires rest and looking after yourself. It is a large operation and the physical and emotional repercussions can take some time to recover from. However, most women report a good recovery from a mastectomy and many are relieved that the site of the cancer is now removed.

Chemotherapy

Chemotherapy is a combination of drugs, usually delivered intravenously (directly into the vein). There are over 50 chemotherapy drugs and the combination you are offered will depend on the size, type and stage of your cancer. The purpose of chemotherapy is to destroy cancer cells.

Because chemotherapy is carried in the blood, it can reach cancer cells anywhere in the body. Healthy cells can repair the damage caused by the chemotherapy drugs, but cancerous cells are unable to do this and die off.

'There are over 50 chemotherapy drugs and the combination you are offered will depend on the size, type and stage of your cancer.'

Chemotherapy affects all the cells in the body and because of this it can cause unpleasant side effects. It is worth remembering that these side effects are temporary – healthy cells will begin to renew themselves as soon as the therapy is over.

Some healthy cells are more sensitive to chemotherapy than others. The most obvious ones for breast cancer patients are the hair follicles. This is why chemotherapy patients can lose their hair during treatment. Other sensitive areas include the lining of the mouth – some chemotherapy patients will suffer from mouth ulcers during treatment.

The digestive system can also be adversely affected, which is why many chemotherapy patients report nausea as a side effect. The bone marrow, which makes red and white blood cells, is also affected and can cause extreme tiredness.

Chemotherapy is given in 'rounds' or cycles, which means a set number of sessions (often six) with rest periods in between for the body to recover.

A common treatment for breast cancer is FEC chemotherapy. FEC are the initials of the three drugs included in the therapy. They are Fluorouracil, Epirubicin and Cyclophosphamide.

It is worth remembering that however severe the symptoms are when undergoing chemotherapy, they will subside as soon as the treatment has finished. Although it can take several months to feel completely well, your body will start repairing itself as soon as the treatment stops.

Radiotherapy

Radiotherapy is very commonly used in the treatment of cancer. It uses high energy x-rays to kill cancer cells in a localised area. Unlike chemotherapy, which travels through the entire system, radiotherapy is specifically targeted at the site of the original cancer.

Although healthy cells can be damaged by radiotherapy, they are usually able to repair themselves, whereas cancer cells cannot and will die.

Radiotherapy can be used on its own or before or after surgery. Occasionally, it is used in conjunction with chemotherapy. Radiotherapy treatment for breast cancer usually involves visiting the hospital every day for anything from between two and seven weeks, depending on the cancer. Because of the size of all the equipment needed, only larger hospitals have radiotherapy units. This may mean that you receive radiotherapy at a different hospital to the initial treatment.

Most people report that the side effects of radiotherapy are quite mild (particularly in comparison with chemotherapy). However, the most commonly reported side effects include tiredness and localised skin reaction.

'Although healthy cells can be damaged by radiotherapy, they are usually able to repair themselves, whereas cancer cells cannot and will die.'

Hormone therapies

There are two female hormones that can affect cancer cells, which are oestrogen and progesterone. Altering the levels of these hormones in the body can have an inhibiting effect on the growth of cancer cells. The type of hormone treatment you might be offered will depend on whether you are post- or pre-menopausal and if the breast cancer cells have oestrogen receptors (ER).

There are two types of hormone treatment. These are:

- Tamoxifen.
- Aromatase inhibitors (e.g. Arimidex).

If you are suitable for hormone therapy, you may be offered it before or after surgery, or if the cancer has returned.

Most usually hormone therapy is administered for five years after the initial cancer treatment.

Tamoxifen

Tamoxifen prevents oestrogen going into breast cancer cells. It helps lower the risk of the cancer recurring and lowers the risk of breast cancer in the other breast by up to 40%. Tamoxifen is most usually used in women who have not yet reached menopause.

Tamoxifen is proven to greatly increase survival rates in women with breast cancer. However, as with all drugs, there are some side effects. Many women report hot flushes while taking the drug, as well as a slower metabolism (leading to weight gain) and loss of libido (sex drive).

Aromatase inhibitors

Aromatase inhibitors are most usually used in women who have reached menopause and have been diagnosed with early stage breast cancer. Usually these drugs are given after surgery and are proven to be very effective in reducing the risk of recurrent breast cancer.

Although post-menopausal women no longer produce oestrogen from their ovaries, the do still produce a small amount via the adrenal gland and these drugs work by blocking its production completely.

Side effects of hormone therapies

Broadly, all hormone therapies have similar side effects with varying degrees of severity.

These can include:

- Hot flushes.
- Mood changes.
- Lack of interest in sex.
- Vaginal dryness.
- Tiredness.

- Nausea.

- Painful joints.

If you experience any of these side effects while taking hormone therapies, there may be ways to minimise them.

You can find out more information on the side effects of hormone treatment for cancer and how to cope with them at www.breastcancer.org. There is a very useful comparison chart in the 'treatment and side effects' section.

Alternative treatments

Some people want to explore the possibility of alternative treatments for cancer. Alternative treatments mean those that are not offered through your doctor or oncologist (a doctor qualified in the treatment of cancer). Some alternative treatments insist on using no conventional medicine, while others believe they can be used in conjunction with conventional treatment.

A word of warning – alternative cancer treatments are big business. There are many, many 'miracle' stories on the Internet and plenty of unscrupulous people willing to prey on the vulnerability of cancer patients. There are also plenty more who undoubtedly have cancer patients' best interests at heart, but it might be difficult to tell the difference!

Alternative treatments are usually unregulated and un-researched (or have minimal research statistics to back up claims). Going down the alternative route is a very personal decision, which needs a lot of careful thought and support.

There is a lot of information on the different types of alternative treatments currently available at www.canceractive.com.

'Going down the alternative route is a very personal decision, which needs a lot of careful thought and support.'

Breast reconstruction

Breast reconstruction surgery is sometimes offered at the same time as a mastectomy (this is referred to as an immediate reconstruction), or, if further treatment is needed (particularly radiotherapy), it may be offered at a later date (this is called a delayed reconstruction). You could also be offered an immediate delayed reconstruction – this is where the breast tissue is conserved at the time of the mastectomy in order for a reconstruction to occur at a later date using the patient's own breast tissue.

Commonly, if there hasn't been an immediate breast reconstruction, the patient may have to wait for up to two years to be offered a reconstruction. This varies according to the policy in your local health authority, or your particular surgeon's preference.

The wait is usually to allow the body to fully heal after treatment and also because the highest rates of recurrence of breast cancer are in the first two years from initial diagnosis. Some doctors feel it is better to wait to ensure that all the possible treatment is finished before embarking on further surgery. There are various types of breast reconstruction surgery and your surgeon will advise which is best for you.

What is breast reconstruction?

Breast reconstruction aims to create a breast mound that is similar in size and shape to the remaining breast or, in the case of a double reconstruction, to mimic how the breasts looked before surgery. However, it is impossible to exactly match the existing breast and if you are considering reconstruction, it may be worth looking at pictures of reconstructed breasts so you have a good idea of what to expect. There are some photos at www.thebreastclinic.co.uk/photos, or your surgeon may have pictures of their own work, which will give you a very good idea of the type of results achieved.

It is also worth remembering that two or three operations may be required to get a good match. The reconstructed breast can be higher, bigger or smaller than the natural breast (particularly if implants have been used). This may mean surgery on the natural breast to reduce, enlarge or lift. This can be done at the same time as the reconstruction, but it is more commonly performed at a later date when the reconstructed breast has settled down.

The reconstructed breast will not have a nipple, although nipple reconstruction can be performed as a separate operation at a later date.

The main benefit of a reconstruction is that a prosthesis is no longer needed. This can be very liberating for a lot of women and means that you can wear 'normal' bras again rather than special post-mastectomy bras with pockets for prosthesis.

Breast reconstruction can also give you a cleavage, which means a wider choice in the type of clothes or swimming costume you can wear. After waiting a long time for a reconstruction, this can be a huge benefit – both psychologically and emotionally.

An immediate reconstruction can lessen the trauma of a mastectomy, as there is no period with a loss of breast shape. However, immediate reconstruction is a longer operation with a longer recovery time and may not be an option for all types and stages of breast cancer.

Types of breast reconstruction

Broadly, there are two types of breast reconstruction – those using implants and those using your own tissue. Reconstruction using your own tissue involves using fat and/or muscle from another area of your body.

Breast reconstruction using implants

Breast reconstruction using implants under the muscle can be done when breast tissue has been removed but the skin (and sometimes the nipple) is kept. The tissue is replaced with an implant. This type of reconstruction is only suitable for women with very early stage breast cancer.

It is not suitable for women who have undergone a radical mastectomy (total removal of the breast and muscles from the chest wall). Some stages and grades of breast cancer require radiotherapy as soon as the mastectomy site has healed and you will not be offered this type of surgery if there is a chance of needing radiotherapy, as the skin covering the breast will not be elastic enough to cope.

Breast reconstruction using tissue expansion

Breast reconstruction using tissue expansion uses the skin's natural ability to stretch to create a new breast. However, this takes several months and again is not suitable if you have had radiotherapy, or might need it in the future.

The most usual method of tissue expansion is an operation to insert an implant that is capable of expansion (rather like a flat balloon). A small valve is placed under the chest muscle and saline solution (salt water) is slowly injected into the implant. This is usually performed weekly or fortnightly to allow the skin to stretch gradually, and it can take several months.

After the breast has achieved its optimum size, a second operation is required to remove the saline implant and replace it with a permanent silicone implant.

Breast reconstruction using flaps

This type of reconstruction uses muscle, tissue, fat and skin (known as flaps) from another area of the body to create a breast shape. This is a major operation, usually requiring a hospital stay of at least one week.

Broadly, there are two types of flap reconstruction. Latissimus dorsi (LD flap) uses a large muscle from your back brought around to the front of the body. Tissue, fat and skin from your own body will be used. Often, a LD reconstruction will also use silicone implants to create as natural a breast shape as possible.

The second common flap reconstruction is called a TRAM flap and uses fat, skin and some muscle from the abdomen. TRAM flaps can create a more natural feeling breast, but it is a much bigger operation with a longer recovery time.

Both operations result in a double scar site. The LD leaves a scar on the back. The surgeon will usually try to ensure that this scar runs under the bra strap line to minimise any visibility. The TRAM flap will leave a long scar on the abdomen. All scars will fade back over time and their appearance can be greatly improved by massaging regularly with moisturiser or oil for the purpose.

Summing Up

- Depending on your individual circumstances, you will be offered treatment for your cancer. This may be surgery, chemotherapy, radiotherapy or hormonal therapy. If you undergo a mastectomy, you will need, at some point, a breast reconstruction operation.

- Understanding treatment, side effects and options can be very confusing. Your doctor may talk to you about certain treatments, but it may not mean much to you at the time. It is only afterwards that you may want to read a little more about the type of treatment you have been offered in order to understand how it works.

- It may feel as though you are on a medical conveyor belt, with one treatment after another. It might feel as if the treatment is never going to end. Some breast cancer treatment can take up to a year from start to finish – it will be a very stressful time for you and your family and it's important that you find a way of coping that suits your individual circumstances.

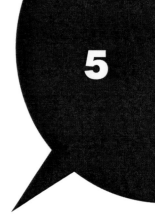

5

Your Feelings and Emotions

How you feel after a cancer diagnosis will largely depend on your stage of life, the severity of the cancer and your general wellbeing before the diagnosis. However, most women will initially experience some form of shock. Nobody wants to hear that they have cancer and it can come as a particular trauma if you are young or fit and healthy and have had no particular symptoms.

Dealing with the shock of diagnosis

Often, when a woman hears the word cancer, she immediately thinks she is going to die. Instead of hearing the words 'We have found cancerous cells', she may hear 'You are going to die of cancer'. This is by no means a certainty. Breast cancer survival rates are improving all the time. Many breast cancer patients will go on to live long, happy and healthy lives. The latest survival statistics are extremely optimistic and are constantly improving.

'Many breast cancer patients will go on to live long, happy and healthy lives. The latest survival statistics are extremely optimistic and are constantly improving.'

However, despite this, any cancer diagnosis can come as a huge shock. Nobody thinks that it will happen to them and any illness means a readjustment of expectations and having to face the trials of treatment.

The first person you might meet after a breast cancer diagnosis is a breast care nurse. These are nurses who are specially trained in all aspects of breast cancer care and will be there to help you through the treatment process. Some people find it easier to ask the breast care nurse questions, as they feel that the doctors are too busy. The breast care nurses work as part of the medical team dealing with your treatment, so they will be aware of the type of cancer you have and your treatment options.

Everyone is different and the support required will vary widely from person to person. However, most people find talking to someone sympathetic can be a great help. This may be someone amongst your friends or family, or it could be a professional who is trained to listen.

Counselling

Often, breast cancer treatment clinics will have counsellors available. It can be extremely useful to talk to someone who is not immediately connected with you. It may be that you want to talk about difficult issues, like 'What will happen if I die?', which are hard to bring up with family members without them becoming upset. Or you may want to express your anger in a safe environment and protect your family from some of your more negative feelings.

Complementary therapies

Complementary therapies are not alternative treatments for cancer, rather they are therapies that can work alongside conventional treatment and may help improve the quality of life for the patient. They include treatments such as:

- Reflexology – the physical act of applying pressure to the feet or hands with specific thumb, finger and hand techniques without the use of oils. It is based on a system of zones that reflect an image of the body on the hands and feet, with the premise that manipulating these areas causes a physical change to the body.

- Massage – the manipulation of muscles and tissues on the body. It usually uses oils or lotions and is primarily used to promote relaxation and wellbeing.

- Hypnotherapy – attempts to address the subconscious mind in order to bring about a change in conscious thinking. For example, hypnotherapy can be used to combat phobias, such as flying or a needle phobia.

- Equine therapy – uses building a relationship with horses in order to overcome fears, build self-confidence, develop trust, increase communication skills and problem solving. The skills learned within the therapy can be transferred to everyday life.

- Acupuncture – uses needles on specific sites of the body in order to promote healing and physical and mental wellbeing. It is based on the theory of good health being inextricably linked with good energy flow through the body. Acupuncture is a very ancient healing tool.

For more information on complementary therapies, please see *Complementary Therapies – The Essential Guide* (Need2Know).

'Complementary therapies are not alternative treatments for cancer, rather they are therapies that can work alongside conventional treatment and may help improve the quality of life for the patient.'

Support groups

Most local health authorities will have breast cancer support groups. There are sometimes separate groups for younger women who have been diagnosed with breast cancer. The first point of contact will be your breast care nurse, who will have all the latest contact details for your local groups.

Online support

There are also many online support groups available for women with breast cancer. Some women are more comfortable using online support. Others, particularly those in very rural areas, might find it easier to access support online than physically making it along to meetings.

Macmillan and Breast Cancer Care both offer excellent online support groups (see help list).

Be kind to yourself

Many women are not very good at getting support for themselves, as they are more used to supporting everyone else. The good news is that there is lot of support available for women with breast cancer.

'Many women are not very good at getting support for themselves, as they are more used to supporting everyone else.'

It is crucially important that you are supported through this time. If you have a partner and/or children, you will have the added stress of coping with their feelings and emotions on top of your own – it can be a very daunting prospect. If you are single and facing a breast cancer diagnosis, you will need to plan your support strategies, either from close friends or family, or perhaps from more formal support groups or professionals in your area.

For some women, having a cancer diagnosis can be the first time they have really put themselves first for years. Although it is important to be aware of others' feelings, it is also vitally important to listen to your own emotions at this time. You may find you instinctively know how best to manage your illness, when to rest or when to seek out company and activity. Listen to yourself as you know your own body best.

Be kind to yourself and don't expect too much. If you are tired, try to rest. If you are sad, find a friend to have a cry with. Try not to become too isolated with your feelings, or feel that you have to become Superwoman coping with everything at once. Let others take some of the strain and don't be afraid to ask for help. Keep a journal if it helps, or take some time to look at beautiful things in art or nature. Nourishing the soul is as important as healing the body.

It can also be very beneficial to factor in some treats during your treatment for breast cancer. It is easier to get through the horrible times if you have something to look forward to. This could be something as small as going to the cinema (maybe in the daytime for extra decadence!) or as big as planning a holiday.

You will have to find your own way to cope with the upheaval of a cancer diagnosis; everyone is different, so have a think and do what is right for you. There are all sorts of options – find a local support group, ask for one-to-one counselling, and spend time doing the things you love. If you love gardening but don't feel well enough to do any, see if you can visit a local garden for inspiration. If you love walking in the countryside but are not up to hiking, see if you can go for a drive somewhere new or different. Modify activities you can't manage and plan for the time when you will be able to enjoy them fully again.

Also, remember that there will be good days and bad days. There will be times when your whole world feels overwhelming. It is okay to have those negative feelings and to rail against your fate. These negative feelings can give you the impetus to get well and find ways to feel better.

Give thanks on the better days.

Communication

A breast cancer diagnosis can leave everyone, not just the patient, feeling fearful and full of questions. When you are the person who has been diagnosed with cancer, it may be difficult to think about other people's feelings because you are so busy coping with your own. Sometimes it can feel as though everyone else has got it easy because they haven't got cancer. However, it is really important to try to keep the lines of communication open with your friends and family and understand that it is difficult for them too.

'However, it is really important to try to keep the lines of communication open with your friends and family and understand that it is difficult for them too.'

The most common feelings after a cancer diagnosis for the patient and their carers are:

- Fear – fear comes in many forms. There is the fear of the future, the fear of the treatment, the fear of pain and the fear of death. Both the patient and the carers will be experiencing these emotions.

- Anger – anger can arise when thinking 'Why me? What have I done to deserve this?' This can apply to the cancer patient, who may be full of questions about why the cancer has occurred. However, it can also apply to the carers who may feel ill equipped to deal with a sick partner.

- Frustration – frustration occurs when the illness prevents people from living a 'normal' life. Hospital treatment can take up a lot of time for both the patient and the carer – getting to and from appointments, sitting in waiting rooms and looking for a place to park at the hospital. All these things can lead to frustration. Treatment for cancer may mean that other activities have to be cancelled or rescheduled, which may be very difficult for everyone concerned.

Some cancer treatments, such as chemotherapy, can go on for weeks or months. There may be a sense that it is never going to end, that the treatment will last forever and normal life will never return. It is important to remember that it will change, no matter how grim it gets.

'It is important to give each other time to say exactly what is on your mind. Good listening has the added advantage of helping to avoid mis-understanding.'

The people who will be looking after you on an everyday basis will inevitably feel very stretched and possibly full of conflicting feelings themselves. Even though they want you to be better, of course, they may feel angry or let down or resentful at being put in the caring role. There is the double aspect of the carers not being able to express these feelings or feeling ashamed of them.

Sometimes it might feel to them as if all the focus is on the person with cancer and there is very little support for the carers.

Being a good listener

The key to good communication is being able to listen. It is very hard to hear what other people are saying when you are more interested in how to navigate your way through the cancer diagnosis. However, learning some listening skills might really help your closest relationships and bring you closer together rather than driving you apart.

Not feeling heard within a relationship can be very damaging, so it is important to give each other time to say exactly what is on your mind. Good listening has the added advantage of helping to avoid misunderstanding.

To listen attentively means keeping a comfortable level of eye contact, facing the person who is speaking and encouraging them to continue by smiling and nodding. The most important aspect of being a good listener is not interrupting the person who is speaking. Try to avoid judging and wait to say your bit until you are sure you have fully understood the point.

Reflecting and summarising lets the speaker know that you have heard and understood what they are saying. For example, if somebody says to you 'I feel absolutely exhausted and I don't know how I'm going to cope with the children tomorrow', reflecting and summarising would be to say to them 'You are really tired and worried about tomorrow'. This shows that you have really listened and can give the other person the opportunity to expand, add or amend the initial statement. Sometimes, all it takes is to be heard.

Try to avoid:

- Thinking about what you are going to say before the person has finished speaking.

- Interrupting unnecessarily.

- Reacting emotionally to what is being said.

- Thinking up a clever counter argument before they have finished speaking.

- Fidgeting and avoiding eye contact.

There are some studies that show that divorce rates can be increased after a diagnosis of cancer (Fred Hutchinson Cancer Research Centre, 2009). This can be due to a large range of factors and is by no means inevitable, but these figures highlight the importance of good communication when faced with challenging times.

Summing Up

- Nobody ever wants to hear a diagnosis of cancer and it can be very easy to assume the worst – cancer survival rates are improving all the time and you should try to stay positive. Of course, everyone's circumstances are different and you need to find your own individual way of coping with a diagnosis, be it through friends and family, support groups or counselling.

- Be kind to yourself – it can be very easy to worry about how partners, family and children are doing during a diagnosis and treatment, but the most important thing is to do what you feel is right. If you are tired, try to rest more, if you are feeling active then do something you enjoy, and most importantly make sure you have some treats to look forward to – no matter how small or big.

- Take others into account. On the flipside, it can be very easy to forget about the stress of what your loved ones will be going through – after all, it is you journeying through the diagnosis and treatment. But it's important to remember your family and friends will also be going through a very stressful period and may also find themselves overwhelmed with emotions.

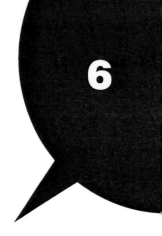

6

Feelings and Emotions of Your Loved Ones

ome women find telling people about their cancer very difficult, while others want to tell everyone immediately. This is a very personal decision. There is no need to tell everyone everything if you don't want to. People can react in extreme ways on hearing about a cancer diagnosis and this can be difficult to cope with on top of the emotions you may be already experiencing. Just saying the words 'I have breast cancer' out loud can be very hard – and you need to feel ready to do this.

Telling your partner

'Some women find telling people about their cancer very difficult, while others want to tell everyone immediately. This is a very personal decision.'

It is likely that the first person to hear the news will be your spouse or partner. The reaction they have, and the support they offer, can be crucial in the treatment journey. Many partners have conflicting emotions when hearing a cancer diagnosis. While they will want to help and do what they can to be supportive, there might also be some fear and resentment there. It is very hard to be ill, but it is also hard to be a caregiver.

Allowing your spouse to be less than perfect, and understanding that they may need support too, can really help. Try to discuss everything in an open and non-judgemental way to avoid emotions being bottled up.

Partners may have very conflicting feelings when faced with a long-term illness. Frustration can play a large part, as can anger and loneliness. It is very important to try to manage these feelings and come to terms with them. Feelings that are unexpressed tend to fester and become worse. If we are allowed to express our feelings, we can usually manage difficult situations much more effectively.

Very often, the caring partner will feel stretched to the limit by all the extra demands made on them. Putting some practical help into place can be very helpful.

Ideas to support your partner

- Respite – it can be a great benefit if the partner who takes on the role of carer has the opportunity to go away for a few days. It is amazing how much a short break can recharge the batteries.

- Relaxation – giving the caring partner regular 'time off' to engage in social activities such as sport or hobbies is very important. Most people can cope if they know there is a window of opportunity for relaxation. It becomes overwhelming or unbearable when a task feels never-ending.

- Support groups – talking to others in a similar situation can really help ease the burden of caring.

- Counselling – the caring partner may feel as though all the focus is on the person who is sick. They may have many feelings they would like to be able to discuss with someone who is a neutral party. For example, they may need a safe environment in which to express their anger about how unfair it all is. Many carers feel they can't do this with their families without looking selfish.

- Help around the house – help with the household chores can really be a lifesaver when everyone is stretched to the limit. If your partner is still working full time, the household chores can just be too much. It is worth remembering that this is a rainy day and all resources need to be put into play. Even if money is tight, it might be worth getting a cleaner while you are undergoing treatment, or perhaps there is a friend or family member who might be happy to help out for a few months. This situation won't last forever, and household help is a short-term solution rather than a long-term drain on the family finances.

Telling children

How and when you tell your children about your breast cancer diagnosis will largely depend on how old they are and if they were aware of any tests you may have had. It is very hard to break the news to children, and they may not react in the way you expect at all. Although there can be general advice about talking to children about a breast cancer diagnosis, how you go about it will be based on your own judgement. No one knows your family and children like you do.

Some experts suggest telling children once you have had time for the news to sink in. If you are tearful and upset, it might be harder for the children to know how to react. This doesn't mean that you can't show or express emotion, it just means being able to focus on the children's needs rather than your own.

You might feel that it is better to tell the whole family together, or each member individually; again this will be largely up to you and how your family cope with traumatic events. Telling the family all together has the advantage of everyone hearing the news at the same time and you not having to repeat it over and over again. Another advantage might be the support of other, older family members such as your parents or siblings. The children will take their cue from how the adults react in this situation and will be looking to the adults to understand how to behave. If you do decide to tell everyone together, make sure that everyone has the time and space to digest the news.

'Feelings that are unexpressed tend to fester and become worse. If we are allowed to express our feelings, we can usually manage difficult situations much more effectively.'

It is up to each family to decide how much or how little to tell children, a lot will depend on their ages and ability to understand, but it is always important to keep them informed of the bigger picture. Children can find secrets particularly difficult to cope with and they need to know that they can trust you to tell them the truth. They may not want to hear every nuance of your treatment, but they will want to be kept informed of how you are getting on. For example, children may not want to hear about the type of drugs you are receiving, but they would understand that Mummy is taking medicine to make her better.

It can come as a shock that children can start to play up just at the time when you need them to be well behaved. The last thing you may need is a child being difficult, but this is what you might get! Try to understand that bad behaviour often arises out of fear and distress, and make an effort not to be too hard on them or yourself. It is important to try to keep the channels of communication open.

'How and when you tell your children about your breast cancer diagnosis will largely depend on how old they are and if they were aware of any tests you may have had.'

What to say?

It is generally agreed that it is better to be honest, straightforward and clear when talking to children about cancer. This doesn't mean frightening them with a barrage of statistics, or being insensitive to their feelings, but it is about being clear about how your cancer diagnosis might affect them.

It is entirely up to you how much detail you want to go into, but it is best not to talk in euphemisms, unless your child/children are very young indeed. For example, if a child asks you if you are going to die, it may be best to face the issue head on. Instead of saying 'No, of course not', it might be better to say something about how the doctors are doing everything they can to make you better and that most women with breast cancer go on to live long and healthy lives.

You may want to talk to the children about what your treatment will involve. How long you will be in hospital, for example, or the effects of chemotherapy. For some children, thought of their mother losing her hair is very frightening, so do stress that any hair loss will be temporary and that it will grow back, even if it looks alarming at the time. Some children will say things like 'You're not going to pick us up from school wearing a wig are you?', which you may feel is a very unfeeling reaction, but being embarrassed in front of their peer group can be of huge importance, especially to young teenagers. Try to talk to them about how you might lessen the embarrassment together. Saying that, they can help choose the wig, or having a range of different wigs to choose from might help alleviate their worries.

Different ages will need a different approach, for example:

- Under threes will have a very limited understanding, but will sense a change in the household routine. It is okay to tell them that Mummy is poorly and that she will need to go to the hospital. Perhaps follow this up with 'So Daddy (or whoever it will be) will be looking after you and you will have lots of fun'.

- Under fives will also want to know who will be looking after them while you are away. They may have a slightly better sense of time, but they won't be able to understand concepts like 'Mummy will be in hospital for a week' –they may ask whoever is looking after them several times a day if it has been a week yet! Keep conversations with this age range very brief and answer any questions that might come up even if they occur at difficult moments.

- Primary school children may have a lot more awareness of cancer, and they might also associate the word cancer with death. It is very important to allay their fears with language they are able to understand. Primary school children will also have a clearer understanding of time, so you can be definite about your treatment and how long it might take; for example, chemotherapy will take five months, radiotherapy will take six weeks. Children will want to be reassured that their activities and daily life will not be too disrupted – so talk to them about plans you will put in place to make sure everything remains as normal as possible.

- Teenagers will have more of an idea of what cancer is and how it can affect people. Teenagers are usually going through a lot of emotional change and difficulty themselves, and you may find that they are very angry about your diagnosis. They may blame you, or feel that bad things only happen to them and their family. They may react in very surprising ways to your diagnosis, often showing quite 'difficult' behaviour. Of course, not all teenagers react this way. Some people find that the opposite is true and their teenage children rise to the challenge and grow up a lot as a result.

'For all children, it is a good idea to let their school or nursery know what is happening at home.'

Schools

For all children, it is a good idea to let their school or nursery know what is happening at home. Even if they appear to be coping, there might be a change in behaviour at school, which could be confusing for teachers who are unaware of the changes. Your child might have an easier time if everyone involved with his or her welfare knows the situation and can make allowances accordingly.

Support for carers

Until recently, most research has been carried out on the effect of a cancer diagnosis on the patient. However, there is now a growing realisation of the effects of cancer on a couple and, by extension, the whole family. The emotional impact on the couple has sparked a whole new area of research. There are some studies that suggest the carer can feel more distress and despair than the person who is sick.

Indeed, a study in the *Journal of Oncology* (Lewis *et al.*, 2008) reported that spouses were lonelier than their ill partners and had lower levels of wellbeing and marital satisfaction. There is an immediate shift in a relationship when an illness is diagnosed; one person becomes more dependent on the other and is less able to contribute to the daily running of the household. This can lead to feelings of fear, not just about the disease, but about the strength of the relationship and the well partner's ability to cope. Feelings of anger and resentment about life and the situation can quickly arise.

There is a lot of adapting within a relationship when a woman gets cancer. The well partner may still be working full time, but with additional demands on their time such as household chores, driving to and from hospital and, crucially, childcare arrangements. Even the most devoted partner could become exhausted. The carer may feel they need support to cope with all these extra tasks.

There is also a difference in how men and women approach problems. For many women, being listened to is the most important aspect. For many men, this is a counter intuitive way of coping with a stressful situation. Their instinct is to want to 'fix' things with a practical solution. They can be so busy trying to run the home and keep everything together that the small things, like a hug, can be overlooked.

Of course, you and your partner need to deal with the situation as best you can – there is much evidence to show that some couples feel closer after weathering such a sudden storm together. It can take time and effort to accept the changes that take place as a result of a breast cancer diagnosis, but many couples do find that their love grows stronger as a result.

Summing Up

- When to tell family and friends is a very personal decision; it can cause people to react in very different ways and only you can know the best way to approach the subject. Perhaps it is better to let the news sink in a bit before breaking the news to others, or perhaps you need that support network in place from the beginning, in which case telling others will be a priority.

- Your partner will probably be the first person you confide in, it will be a very difficult time and sometimes things can get too much. Be kind to your partner and allow some time for relaxation and respite. Try to come up with practical ways to overcome the obstacles that daily life throws at you both.

- Breaking the news to your children will be a very emotional but necessary task – try to word it in a way appropriate to their age and don't be surprised if they react in an inappropriate or selfish way. Fear and distress will often breed this kind of reaction.

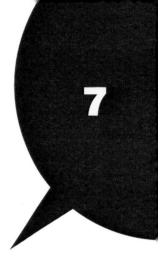

7

The Road to Recovery

Diet

Many people radically change their diet after a breast cancer diagnosis. There have been several studies linking diet and breast cancer, and many books have been written about managing breast cancer through diet.

However, changing your diet is controversial. There are studies that disagree with extreme diet changes. Make sure you speak to your doctor before making any extreme dietary changes, as it could have an adverse effect on your health.

'Cutting down on high-fat, high-sugar foods and increasing fresh fruit and vegetables are all part of a healthy eating approach.'

Women can be prone to feeling guilty around food – and following an extreme diet can increase these feelings of guilt. For example, if you don't manage to keep to the rigid eating rules or slip on some days, you may experience low self-esteem, which isn't good for mental health. While it is clearly a good idea to eat sensibly and think about ways of tweaking or modifying your diet to ensure you get the best nutrition, it might also be a good idea not to be too rigid about it. Cutting down on high-fat, high-sugar foods and increasing fresh fruit and vegetables are all part of a healthy eating approach.

Many women, however, feel that diet is one thing they can control. When breast cancer strikes, it is very hard to know how to help yourself and modifying your diet can help towards regaining some control over your body and a feeling that you are doing the best for your recovery.

It appears to make logical sense that a healthy diet will result in a healthy body. There are studies linking breast cancer and being overweight, so keeping within a healthy BMI is a good idea. There are several common diet changes that some women have found beneficial, some of which are listed overleaf.

Going dairy free

You don't have to look very far to find articles about the link between dairy foods and breast cancer. As just mentioned, these links are controversial, but there are many women who believe that cutting out dairy can help in the fight against breast cancer.

The World Cancer Research Fund does not recommend completely cutting dairy from your diet. However, it does recommend choosing low-fat varieties, such as semi-skimmed milk and low-fat yoghurt, as a way of limiting animal fats. Eating a plant-based diet is proven to be healthier in the fight against cancer.

Dairy is a good source of protein, calcium, vitamin B12 and riboflavin. It is possible to get these from other sources such as green leafy vegetables (for example, broccoli, chard and cabbage), pulses (including soya products like tofu and soya milk) and some nuts such as almonds, hazelnuts and Brazil nuts.

Vegetable juicing

The arguments for vegetable juicing and its health benefits are many and varied. Even though most people are aware of the need to eat at least five portions of fresh vegetables and fruit per day, not many people actually manage it. In fact, one American study (Kimmonds *et al.*, 2009) showed that the average adult ate only one-and-a-half portions of vegetables per day and no fruit at all. Five portions are considered the absolute minimum – and some experts recommend up to nine portions per day to ensure health giving benefits.

Vegetable juicing is one way to increase your daily intake. However, vegetable juicing machines can be expensive and it is quite a commitment to juice every day. Also, some people don't like the taste or texture of vegetable juice. On the plus side, if you are finding it difficult to reach the recommended portions of fruit and vegetables per day, juicing might help boost your target.

If you think you might like to try juicing, there are many books available. There are also many websites devoted to raw foods and juicing, with free recipes available to all. Although juicing is not proven to help in the fight against cancer, it may help increase your five a day target in order to maintain optimum health.

There are some vegetable juices that can be made in a blender and it might be an idea to start with those and see how you get on before investing in an expensive juicer.

Beta-Carrot Juice

Ingredients

2 apples
½ beetroot
2 small carrots
1 small parsnip
¼ lemon (unwaxed if possible, with the skin on)
Ice

Method

1 Chop the ingredients into cubes or slices.

2 Juice the apples, beetroot, carrots, parsnip and lemon (pack the lemon between the other produce).

3 Pour over ice.

Spinach Stout

Ingredients

2 large handfuls of baby spinach
¼ pineapple
¼ cucumber
1 medium carrot
½ lemon, peeled
Ice

Method

1 Chop the ingredients into cubes or slices.

2 Juice the spinach, pineapple, cucumber, carrot and lemon by packing the spinach and lemon between the other produce.

3 Pour over ice.

Carrot 'n' Pineapple Twist

Ingredients

2 carrots
¼ pineapple
¼ lemon (unwaxed with the skin on)
Ice

Method

1 Chop the ingredients into cubes or slices.

2 Juice the carrots, pineapple and lemon by packing the lemon between the other produce.

3 Pour over ice.

Vitamins

The use of high doses of vitamins to fight cancer is very controversial. The best way to get the vitamins your body needs is through a balanced diet.

There is a tendency to think of vitamins and vitamin supplements as being 'natural' and therefore harmless in the worse-case scenario and beneficial in the best. This is not always the case. Some high doses of vitamins can interfere with the effectiveness of cancer treatments like chemotherapy and radiotherapy.

Currently, there is no solid evidence that high doses of vitamins can help fight cancer. The Royal College of Radiologists (2006) specifically advise against taking high antioxidant supplements, such as selenium, co-enzyme Q10 and the vitamins A, C and E, while receiving radiotherapy. It is apparent that there needs to be a lot more research in this area.

Mostly doctors will only advise taking a vitamin supplement if there is a proven lack of a particular vitamin in a patient; for example, in cases of anaemia (lack of iron) or if HRT is weakening the bones (lack of calcium). In those cases, iron or calcium and vitamin D might be prescribed. If a patient is unable, due to medical reasons, to absorb vitamins from a normal diet, then a single good-quality, multivitamin may be advised. If you feel that you would like to take dietary supplements, it would be worthwhile talking to you doctor or oncologist about how effective they might be.

The best way of ensuring adequate supplies of vitamins and minerals is through a healthy diet.

'Some high doses of vitamins can interfere with the effectiveness of cancer treatments like chemotherapy and radiotherapy.'

Meat

The link between eating meat and an increase in cancer risk raises some questions. Firstly, there appears to be a difference between processed meat products, such as burgers, sausages, salami, etc, and lean cuts of meat, which has no association with cancer (Thorogood, 1994).

It has been proven that processed meats do have the potential to increase cancer risk slightly, particularly bowel cancer. Red meat has also been cited as increasing cancer risk. One study by the Archives of Internal Medicine (Eunyoung et al., 2006) found that high red meat consumption was linked to hormone receptor positive breast cancer. Hormone receptor positive breast cancer means that the tumour is oestrogen-receptor positive (ER Positive). This means it is more likely to grow in a high oestrogen environment.

As in all dietary advice, moderation appears to be the key. The study that proved a link between red meat and certain types of breast cancer showed that it was women who ate more than one-and-a-half portions per day. A portion was considered to be a hamburger-sized helping. Women who ate three or less servings per week had a lower incidence of breast cancer.

Lean cuts of meat include chicken breast, turkey, and fish.

Fat

Eating a diet high in fat is proven to increase the risk of certain cancers, particularly breast cancer (National Research Council, 1989). However, it is important to be aware of the different types of fat we eat and why our bodies require certain types of fat in order to stay healthy.

Broadly, there are saturated, monounsaturated and polyunsaturated fat. The fat that has been shown to increase incidents of breast cancer (especially in post-menopausal women) is saturated fat. The types of food that are high in saturated fat are full-fat dairy products (such as cheese, cream and butter) and fatty red meat.

'As in all dietary advice, moderation appears to be the key.'

Monounsaturated fats are found in oils, such as olive oil. Olive oil contains monounsaturated fat which protects levels of 'good' cholesterol (important for heart health and function) while reducing 'bad' cholesterol. However, olive oil is still very high in calories, so if you are trying to reduce your weight, be aware that there are a similar amount of calories in olive oil as in butter or lard.

Polyunsaturated fats are further classified into two groups – omega 3 and omega 6.

Omega 6 fats are found in foods such as sunflower margarine. Although less damaging than saturated fats, they are not as beneficial as monounsaturated fats. They have been shown to help reduce total cholesterol; however, at the same time they can also reduce the 'good' cholesterol – which is an adverse effect.

Omega 3 fats are found in foods such as oily fish like pilchards, sardines and trout. Omega 3 is also found in some seeds and nuts, such as linseed and walnuts. Omega 3 fats do not directly affect cholesterol levels, but they have been shown to help reduce the chances of forming blood clots.

Having two small portions of oily fish a week should ensure an adequate intake of omega 3 oils. Furthermore, due to evidence that oily fish has high mercury content, it is recommended by the Food Standards Agency that no more than two portions per a week are eaten and that pregnant women should only have one portion per week.

Exercise

As part of a recipe for a healthier lifestyle, regular exercise has to play a very important role. Exercise helps control weight, makes the body physically stronger and greatly improves psychological and emotional wellbeing.

Regular exercise is considered to be 30-45 minutes of moderate exercise at least five times per week. Moderate exercise can include brisk walking, carrying heavy shopping, gardening and even some forms of housework. As a general rule, moderate exercise should leave you slightly out of breath but able to carry on a conversation (although perhaps not able to sing a song!).

Vigorous exercise includes activities like running, cycling, swimming, lifting weights or an exercise class. Vigorous exercise means that you would not be able to carry on a conversation while you are exercising.

Exercise and breast cancer

If there is one thing you remember after reading this book, hopefully it is this: regular, moderate exercise can decrease the incidence of secondary cancer by 50% (Holmes *et al.*, 2005). This is higher than any drug treatment currently available.

If a drug company managed to develop a pill that reduced the recurrence rates of cancer by 50%, it would be considered a huge breakthrough in the battle against cancer. The drug company would be on course to make millions of pounds and most patients would be prepared to pay for the chance of such a good outcome. Taking up walking or running requires very little equipment. Some health authorities will subsidise gym membership for certain patients (it is always worth asking).

'Regular, moderate exercise can decrease the incidence of secondary cancer by 50%. This is higher than any drug treatment currently available.'

Exercise support

Starting to take exercise after a cancer diagnosis can be a very daunting prospect, particularly if you feel overweight or your body image has been shaken by surgery. It can be very helpful to exercise with other women in the same situation. There are a few places in the UK that run exercise programmes specifically for breast cancer patients. Lobbying for more access to exercise opportunities for women recovering from breast cancer has to be very important.

Taking regular exercise is a habit that can boost your chances of beating cancer by a significant degree. Although it is very hard to get motivated, regular exercise appears to be the most effective and proven way of combating many different types of cancer.

To find out more about exercising after a cancer diagnosis, the not-for-profit organisation the National Association of Cancer Exercise Rehabilitation has many inspiring facts and stories. Visit www.nacer.org.uk.

Macmillan also has some very good information on its website about exercise before, during and after a cancer diagnosis.

Fatigue

Cancer related fatigue is a very real issue for some cancer patients. Many people report a loss of energy and an impairment of physical performance after a cancer diagnosis and treatment. Some researchers estimate that this problem affects up to 70% of cancer patients during chemotherapy and radiotherapy or after surgery. Furthermore, up to 30% of cancer survivors have been reported to experience a loss of energy for years after treatment has finished (Dimeo *et al.,* 1997).

For many patients, this is a severe and life-limiting symptom. This impairment in physical fitness is a significant contributor to decreased quality of life. In response to fatigue, patients are often advised to rest and reduce their level of daily activities. But since inactivity induces weakening of the muscles, prolonged rest can actually perpetuate fatigue.

Aerobic exercise (defined as the rhythmical contraction and relaxation of large muscle groups over a prolonged time) has been suggested for rehabilitation of cancer patients affected by fatigue. Many cancer patients and some doctors believe that vigorous exertion is potentially harmful, although no evidence supports this notion. On the contrary, there is a growing body of evidence that shows exercise improves the physical performance of cancer patients.

Wellbeing

Wellbeing, or quality of life, is difficult to define and difficult to measure. This is because it can mean different things to different people. The simplest definition of quality of life is the degree to which a person enjoys his or her life.

A more detailed definition of quality of life can be split into three areas: 'being', 'belonging' and 'becoming'.

Being includes the 'physical being'. This is our nutrition and exercise requirements, as well as being able to physically get around. Also in this category is 'psychological being', which includes being free of worry and stress and the overall mood a person is in. 'Spiritual being' is defined as having hope for the future and a 'moral compass', or clear idea of right and wrong.

Belonging includes 'physical belonging' – that is, the house or flat in which you live and the geographical area it is in. 'Social belonging' includes family, being in a relationship or having a wide circle of friends. 'Community belonging' would include having access to healthcare services and having enough money for your needs.

Becoming refers to purposeful activities carried out to achieve personal goals, hopes or wishes. 'Practical becoming' describes day-to-day activities like domestic duties or work. 'Leisure becoming' includes activities to promote relaxation and reduce stress. This could be walking the dog or belonging to a group that promotes a particular hobby. 'Growth becoming' means the capacity to build on skills, reach improvement goals and having a framework with which to cope with change.

Some studies show that breast cancer patients who do not experience a recurrence of their cancer are equally as happy as women who haven't had cancer at all, when polled eight years after diagnosis (Dorval et al., 1998). Anecdotally, many women report that a breast cancer diagnosis has made them rethink how they are living their lives, ensuring they make more time for the things that are important to them. There are some women who radically alter their lives after a breast cancer diagnosis.

Many women report a breast cancer diagnosis as being a 'wake-up call'; a reminder that life is short and should be lived to the full. For others though, a serious illness can lead to depression and low self-esteem. If you are experiencing frequent low mood, it is definitely worth talking to your doctor about it. There are many ways in which they can help. The first step is to identify how you are feeling and which areas you feel could improve. This will help your doctor to know what would be best for you and to help you both decide on a course of treatment.

Time to reflect

A breast cancer diagnosis makes many women reflect on their life and choices. Some feel that they want to make changes in how they live their life. This could mean making dietary changes, taking up regular exercise, spending more time doing enjoyable hobbies or making the time to be with friends and family.

There are a minority of people who make radical changes to their lifestyle by training for a new career, for example, or taking steps to fulfil a lifelong dream. Many women who have been through the breast cancer experience will say that they have become very aware of how precious life is and they feel they haven't a moment to lose. They also report wanting to be in control of their life rather than feeling victim to fate.

For others, the stress and physical impact of the diagnosis can leave them feeling very low and out of control of their bodies and lives. How each individual woman reacts will depend on individual circumstances.

'Many women who have been through the breast cancer experience will say that they have become very aware of how precious life is and they feel they haven't a moment to lose.'

Summing Up

- There are some extreme approaches to diet and a lot of conflicting information – it appears that moderation may be the key. Try to keep to a healthy diet with plenty of fruits and vegetables.

- Exercise seems to be extremely beneficial after a breast cancer diagnosis has been made, reducing your risk of further breast cancer by 50%. Again, try to do things in moderation – if you are suffering from fatigue, don't try to do too much; listen to your body but bear in mind the effectiveness of maintaining an active lifestyle.

- Wellbeing relates to many different aspects of life and is dependent on each person and their circumstances. Do things you enjoy to increase your wellbeing and quality of life.

- Take some time to reflect – many women want to change their lifestyles and attitudes after a breast cancer diagnosis. Do what is right for you and your circumstances.

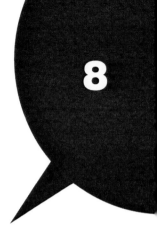

8

Life After Breast Cancer

Emotional effects

We have discussed some of the emotional effects of breast cancer in the previous chapter. How each woman feels after their treatment is over and 'normal' life has resumed will vary from person to person. Every woman who has been through breast cancer will have a different story to tell. No two people will have exactly the same experience, even if they had exactly the same type of cancer and subsequent treatment. The emotional journey through breast cancer is unique to the person going through it.

Some advice you may read about coping with a diagnosis will appear particularly pertinent, while other advice won't be relevant at all. If there is a common thread that links all women who have had breast cancer, it might be the increased ability to listen to themselves and their bodies.

There are women who feel more empowered because of this. They feel less likely to put up with second best or do things they don't want to do. There are many, many support groups, both real and virtual. The Internet is full of breast cancer stories and women wanting to share them. Lots of people feel that writing down their experience is incredibly helpful. Also, many women take comfort in the fact that others may be helped by their experiences. Some women volunteer to become a 'breast cancer buddy' and will support another woman going through the process, either practically or via telephone or email.

For some women, however, it takes a long time to regain their confidence and *joie de vivre* after breast cancer. The trauma of diagnosis and subsequent treatment can stay with them and they may find it difficult to move on. Many women also feel continually anxious that the cancer might return. Also, stories about amazing women who have done incredible things after breast cancer, such as running a marathon or starting a charity, can make them feel worse. Instead of feeling empowered or inspired by these stories, they feel that they could never hope to live up to such lofty ideals.

Some women feel that they are unable to cope with the rigours of the world of work after breast cancer. They may find that pressure and stress is particularly difficult to cope with. Instead of getting back out into the world, they may want to retreat into home life.

The important thing to remember is that there is no right or wrong way to live life after breast cancer. It is your life and up to you how you live it. Although climbing mountains and running races might do it for some people, others might just take pride in their garden, walking the dogs or baking a great cake!

Most women will agree that having breast cancer has changed them on some level. Some changes are positive and some not so positive. There is something to be said about trying to focus on the positive changes and building on the areas that have improved, while trying to minimise the negative effects. Try to address the less positive areas one at a time rather than feeling overwhelmed by the whole.

Practicalities

Work

The cancer charity Macmillan has recently undertaken research that shows that a lot of post-cancer patients experience difficulties returning to work or finding suitable employment. They have identified a range of problems surrounding returning to work and feel that many people aren't getting the right kind of advice and support in this area.

Returning to work after cancer treatment can be very daunting. Some people will want carry on working through their diagnosis and treatment, but most people will need some time off, for recovery after chemotherapy, for example. Extensive time off can make it very difficult to return to work. Some employers may be reluctant to renew contracts after a cancer diagnosis. Even those who have managed to work during treatment may find that they aren't able to cope with the same workload as before. Macmillan has some excellent publications in this area, as well as advisors with up-to-date information who may be able to help with specific queries from both employees and employers. There is also a section on employee's rights, which is well worth a read.

'The important thing to remember is that there is no right or wrong way to live life after breast cancer. It is your life and up to you how you live it.'

Money

Work and money are inextricably linked for most people. If your ability to work is impaired by the physical effects of your cancer then you may qualify for some benefits. However, there are some post-cancer conditions, such as fatigue and low self-esteem, that are difficult to diagnose and won't warrant a sick note from your doctor or oncologist. This can be very frustrating, as most women want to feel like useful members of society again but can't cope with the demands of a full-time job.

Sometimes returning to work on a part-time basis may be the solution, or discussing with your employer about ways to work flexibly. For example, you may know that you are better in the mornings and get tired after lunchtime. It is definitely worth talking to colleagues and bosses about this rather than battling on.

However, working part time means bringing in less money and many people experience financial difficulties after a cancer diagnosis. Again, Macmillan is the first place to go for support and advice.

Travel

'Keeping clear channels of communication open is vital when dealing with relationship issues. If people feel they can't talk about their fears, sadness or loneliness, these feelings often grow and fester.'

There are practical aspects of dealing with life after cancer which need to be considered. Travel insurance is one area that can become trickier, usually becoming more expensive. You may be required to answer a series of questions relating to your cancer and treatment that may feel invasive and rude. Sometimes you are able to exclude your pre-existing medical condition (such as breast cancer) from your travel insurance quote in order to get it cheaper. However, this means that any treatment relating to your breast cancer while aboard will not be covered.

There are companies that deal specifically with insurance for breast cancer patients (see help list) and it is definitely worth shopping around for the best deal. You may find it easier to get travel insurance for Europe than places further afield. It is also worth noting that medical treatment in North America is astronomically expensive, so having proper travel insurance should be a priority in that area.

There is some evidence that women taking Tamoxifen are more susceptible to deep vein thrombosis (DVT), which can occur on long-haul flights. Without specialist cover, insurance companies would refuse to pay out for treatment for this condition, as it is directly linked to breast cancer.

Relationships

Cancer doesn't just affect one person – it affects couples, families and friends. Most women would agree that cancer changes the way you relate to others and, equally importantly, the way they relate to you. Keeping clear channels of communication open is vital when dealing with relationship issues. If people feel they can't talk about their fears, sadness or loneliness, these feelings often grow and fester. Unexpressed feelings lead to unhappiness and isolation.

Partners

Some couples find that a cancer diagnosis makes them realise how much they love each other and how important the relationship is. Cancer can cause everyone to re-evaluate their priorities and, in the best case scenario, everyone is more appreciative of what they have. However, for some couples the opposite is the case. This is particularly true for those who have been experiencing problems before diagnosis. Cancer diagnosis and treatment is undeniably stressful – and stress on top of existing problems can prove significantly detrimental.

It is almost certain that the relationship will experience changes. There will be changes in responsibilities, changes in roles and, of course, changes of needs. Both partners may need more reassurance and patience at this time.

The other major change for some couples is how they think about the future. Cancer can drastically change the hopes and dreams of a partnership. Long-term plans can become very unsecure and couples can feel trapped in dealing with the immediate treatment. This can cause resentment and despair, especially if there are things you have been planning together. It might be helpful to look again at those plans and see what can be salvaged, what can be put on hold and what can be changed to accommodate the new situation.

Friendships

For many people, the thought of cancer and of someone they care about being ill is very frightening. People deal with this in very different ways. Some people want to be caring and nurturing and others find it very difficult to know how to help.

'Often friends will be looking for you to take the lead in bringing up the subject of cancer. They might not want to bring it up for fear of upsetting you.'

Many people have little experience with life-threatening illnesses and may not know what to say or how to act when someone has cancer. Your illness may be frightening, because it is a reminder that cancer can happen to anyone. Some people may have lost a loved one to cancer and your diagnosis may bring up painful memories. For these reasons, some of your friends or family may not be able to offer you the support you expected. Although this is painful, try to remember that their reactions are not a reflection of how much they care about you. While some friends and family may distance themselves from you, others will surprise you with emotional and physical support throughout your illness. Be prepared for your friendships to change.

Often friends will be looking for you to take the lead in bringing up the subject of cancer. They might not want to bring it up for fear of upsetting you. Don't think they are ignoring your illness – they might just be trying to be sensitive. On the flip side, some friends may talk about cancer all of the time and you might find you just want to do 'normal' things with them instead. 'I'm having a day off from cancer today!', is one way of saying it.

Do let friends help if they want to. Helping others makes people feel good about themselves and you are giving them an opportunity to feel useful and wanted. It might help to give specific people specific tasks that they feel comfortable with. For example, the dog walked by your doggy friend, a cake baked by your friend who loves cooking.

Try to stay involved with any social activities you were involved with before diagnosis. You may find invitations to parties or social events stop coming as people assume you won't want to go out, but even if you don't feel up to it when the day arrives, it is nice to be asked. Ask a friend to keep you in the social loop where possible. Do make sure people are aware that you may have to cancel at the last moment if you are not well enough to attend.

Children

Relationships with your children are inevitably going to alter. We have already looked at discussing your diagnosis with the children, but how your relationship might change is a different aspect. Parenting is hard at the best of times; it is particularly hard when you are undergoing treatment for cancer.

Young children may be more needy than usual and older children and teenagers may be more challenging. They will need plenty of reassurance that they will always be cared for and that you will always love them. You may find that help with childcare is very important at this time, but try to stick to the routines and schedules they are used to. Keeping home life as calm and normal as possible is the best way forward.

There is a brilliant book for friends, families and cancer sufferers called *What Can I Do to Help: 75 Practical Ideas for Family and Friends* from Cancer's Frontline by Deborah Hutton. It is packed full of useful and practical ideas for supporting someone who is ill.

Sexuality

It can be very difficult to talk openly about sex, even with a trusted partner. The physical and emotional effects of cancer and cancer treatments often do affect sexuality, even if only temporarily. Fatigue, depression and vaginal dryness can contribute to lowering the desire for sex.

Regaining a satisfactory sex life after cancer can be a challenge, but it is not impossible. It is possibly an area that needs more research and support.

Many women find that taking things slowly and removing the pressure for sex is very helpful. That is, finding intimacy in other ways such as kissing and cuddling can lead to rekindling feelings of closeness with your partner.

Altered body image is also cited as a reason for women to not feel as sexual as they did before. A mastectomy is a removal of a sexual organ and it isn't surprising that it will affect sexuality. However, having a mastectomy doesn't necessarily mean a drop in sexuality. Most women will agree that the biggest sex organ is the mind and if a woman feels loved and cherished, regardless of physical appearance, she is more likely to be sexually responsive.

Breastcancer.org has some very helpful advice on managing sexuality after breast cancer. It can help a lot to know that you are not alone with these feelings and that there are many symptoms that are common to breast cancer survivors and ways to address them

'Regaining a satisfactory sex life after cancer can be a challenge, but it is not impossible. It is possibly an area that needs more research and support.'

Summing Up

- Dealing with the emotional effects of a cancer diagnosis will be individual to each person – do what you feel is best for you and your situation.

- Returning to work can be a struggle for many women after breast cancer – be open and honest with your employers. If you are in any doubt about your rights, give the Macmillan helpline a call. Money can also be a struggle, particularly if you do not go back to full-time work – again, Macmillan can help you find out if you're entitled to any benefits (see help list).

- Depending on your circumstances, relationships may change – so do what you feel is right regarding partners, friends and children. Nobody can know your individual needs regarding this.

- It can be difficult to return to an active sex life – confidence, mind-set and body image have such an effect. Try to take things slowly and if you're not ready, substitute sex with other forms of intimacy like kissing and cuddling. Again, only you can know your own individual needs regarding this.

Help List

Breastcancer.org

Address: Breastcancer.org 120 East Lancaster Avenue Suite 201 Ardmore, PA 19003

Tel: (610) 642 6550

Website: http://www.breastcancer.org/

Info: Breastcancer.org are a large American charity. They will not answer individual queries, but have an FAQ page on their website, as well as free booklets to download and print.

Breast Cancer Care

Address: Breast Cancer Care, Chester House, 1–3 Brixton Road, London, SW9 6DE

Tel: 0808 800 6000

Email: info@breastcancercare.org.uk

Website: https://www.breastcancercare.org.uk/

Info: Breast Cancer Care provides information on breast cancer, fundraising, and caring for loved ones or relatives.

Breast Cancer Now

Address: Breast Cancer Now, 5th Floor, Ibex House, 42 - 47 Minories, London, EC3N 1DY

Tel: 0333 20 70 300

Contact form: http://breastcancernow.org/about-us/got-a-question/contact-us

Website: http://breastcancernow.org/

Info: Breast Cancer Now are the UK's largest breast cancer research charity.

Breast Cancer Support

Address: Breast Cancer Support, Office 185, 88 Lower Marsh, London, SE1 7AB

Tel: 0300 80 80 900

Contact form: http://breastcancersupport.org.uk/contact

Website: http://breastcancersupport.org.uk/

Info: Breast Cancer Support is a UK charity providing care, and helping people with breast cancer in poverty stricken countries who can't afford medication or treatment.

Cancer Active

Address: CANCERactive, Appletree Cottage, Hay Lane, Fulmer, Bucks, SL3 6HJ
Tel: 0300 365 3015
Email: admin@canceractive.com; wendy@canceractive.com
Website: http://www.canceractive.com/
Info: Cancer Active are a small UK charity devoted to empowering cancer sufferers to increase their personal odds of beating the disease. Their website also has a shop.

Cancer Research UK

Address: Cancer Research UK, Angel Building, 407 St John Street, London, EC1V 4AD
Tel: 020 7242 0200
Contact form: https://www.cancerresearchuk.org/about-us/contact-us/submit-a-question
Website: http://www.cancerresearchuk.org/
Info: Cancer Research UK are one of the leading UK fundraisers for cancer. Their website offers many useful resources, as well as information on how to get involved with fundraising.

Health Central

Address: 750 Third Avenue, 6th Floor New York, NY 10017
Tel: (212) 695-2223
Contact form: http://www.remedyhealthmedia.com/content/contact-us
Website: http://www.healthcentral.com/
Info: Health Central is a general interest healthy living website run by Remedy Health Media.

Insure Pink

Address: Insure Pink, Rosalind Franklin House, Oaks Business Park, Fordham Road, Newmarket, CB8 7XN
Tel: 0844 800 0615
Website: http://www.insurepink.co.uk/
Info: Insure Pink are an insurance company with a difference. For every policy taken out, they donate a set amount to the Pink Ribbon Foundation.

MacMillan

Address: Macmillan Cancer Support, 89 Albert Embankment, London, SE1 7UQ
Tel: 0808 808 00 00
Contact form: http://www.macmillan.org.uk/aboutus/contactus/askmacmillanform.aspx
Website: https://www.macmillan.org.uk/
Info: MacMillan are a leading cancer support charity in the UK, and their website offers access to useful information on various forms of cancer as well as fundraising.

NHS Breast Cancer Screening Program

Website: http://www.nhs.uk/Conditions/breast-cancer-screening/Pages/Introduction.aspx
Info: Carries information on breast cancer as well as the services provided by the NHS. Has a search function to find breast cancer screening services in your area here: http://www.nhs.uk/Service-Search/Breast-screening-services/LocationSearch/325

The Breast Clinic

Address: 47 Park Road, London, TW12 1HX
Tel: +44 (0)207 935 2021
Contact form: http://www.thebreastclinic.co.uk/book-appointment
Website: http://www.thebreastclinic.co.uk/
Info: The Breast Clinic is for reconstructive surgery after breast cancer, and is run by Giles Davies, oncoplastic breast surgeon.

The European Prospective Investigation into Cancer and Nutrition

Email: epic@iarc.fr
Website: http://epic.iarc.fr/
Info: EPIC was designed to investigate the relationships between diet, nutritional status, lifestyle and environmental factors and the incidence of cancer and other chronic diseases. EPIC is a large study of diet and health having recruited over half a million (520,000) people in 10 European countries: Denmark, France, Germany, Greece, Italy, The Netherlands, Norway, Spain, Sweden and the United Kingdom.

The Haven

Address: Effie Road, London, SW6 1TB
Tel: 020 7384 0099
Email: london@breastcancerhaven.org.uk
Website: http://www.thehaven.org.uk/
Info: Breast Cancer 'Havens' offer free support for sufferers with no need for a referral. Each visitor to Breast Cancer Haven can expect to receive up to ten free hours of therapy, and friends and family are welcome too. There are locations throughout the UK- the contact information here is for their London branch.

Wear It Pink

Tel: 0800 107 3104
Contact form: http://wearitpink.org/contact/
Website: http://wearitpink.org/about/breast-cancer-awareness-month/
Info: Wear It Pink is a breast cancer charity, who in October (Breast Cancer Awareness Month) encourage people to wear something pink to raise awareness, and donate if possible.

World Cancer Research Fund

Address: 22 Bedford Square, Fitzrovia, London WC1B 3HH
Tel: 0207 343 4200
Email: wcrf@wcrf.org
Website: https://www.wcrf-uk.org/
Info: The WCRF are similar to Cancer Research UK and others. They help sufferers and family through hard times, and raise money towards a cure.

Book List

Breast Cancer for Dummies
By Ronit Elk, John Wiley & Sons, USA, 2003.

Breast Cancer Husband: How to Help Your Wife (and Yourself) Through Diagnosis, Treatment and Beyond
By Marc A Silver, Rodale Press, USA, 2005.

Breast Cancer: The Complete Guide
By Yashaur Hirshaut, Bantam Books Inc., N.Y. USA, 2008.

Complementary Therapies – The Essential Guide
By Antonia Chitty and Victoria Dawson, Need2Know, Peterborough, 2011.

Emotional Support Through Breast Cancer
By Cordelia Galgut, Taylor & Francis, London, 2014.

Food for Health – The Essential Guide
By Sara Kirkham, Need2Know, Peterborough, 2010.

Sexuality and Fertility After Cancer
By Leslie R Schover, John Wiley and Sons, Chichester, 1997.

The Breast Cancer Survivor's Fitness Plan: A Doctor-Approved Workout Plan For a Strong Body and Lifesaving Results
By Carolyn M. Kaelin, McGraw Hill Educational, London, 2006.

The Complete Natural Medicine Guide to Breast Cancer
By Sat Dharam Kaur, Robert Rose Inc., Willowdale, CA, 2004.

What Can I Do to Help: 75 Practical Ideas for Family and Friends from Cancer's Frontline
By Deborah Hutton, Short Books Ltd, London, 2005.

References

Breakthrough Breast Cancer, *Breast Cancer Risk: The Facts Obesity*, Breakthrough Breast Cancer, London, 2006.

CancerHelp UK, *Definite Breast Cancer Risks*, 2010, www.cancerhelp.org.uk/type/breast-cancer/about/risks/definite-breast-cancer-risks#history, accessed 23 July 2010.

Cancer Research UK, *Alcohol and Breast Cancer*, 2009, www.cancerhelp.org.uk/about-cancer/cancer-questions/alcohol-and-breast-cancer, accessed 23 July 2010.

Cancer Research UK, *Cancer Stats: Key Facts Breast Cancer*, 2010, http://info.cancerresearchuk.org/cancerstats/types/breast/, accessed 23 July 2010.

Dimeo *et al.*, *Aerobic exercise as therapy for cancer fatigue [Clinical Sciences: Clinical Investigations]*, Department of Rehabilitation, Prevention and Sports Medicine and Department of Haematology and Oncology, Freiburg, 1997.

Dorval, M *et al.*, 'Long-term quality of life after breast cancer: comparison of 8-year survivors with population controls', *Journal of Clinical Oncology*, 1998, vol. 16, pages 487-94.

Duffy, S *et al.*, 'Absolute numbers of lives saved and over diagnosis in breast cancer screening, from a randomized trial and from the Breast Screening Programme in England', *J Med Screen*, 2010, vol. 17, 25-30. DOI: 10.1258/jms.2009.009094.

Eunyoung, C *et al.*, 'Red meat intake and risk of breast cancer among pre-menopausal women', *Archives of Internal Medicine*, 2006, vol. 166, pages 2253-59.

European Prospective Investigation of Cancer (EPIC), http://www.srl.cam.ac.uk/epic//, accessed 14 Oct 2010.

Fred Hutchinson Cancer Research Centre, *Hereditary Breast and Ovarian Cancer, Past, Present and Future*, Fred Hutchinson Cancer Research Centre, Seattle, 2009.

Furberg H *et al.*, 'Lactation and breast cancer risk', *International Journal of Epidemiology*, 1999, vol. 28, pages 396-402.

Holmes *et al.*, 'Physical activity and survival after breast cancer diagnosis', *Journal of the American Medical Association*, 2005, vol. 293, issue 20, pages 2479-86.

IARC, *7th Handbook on Cancer Prevention*, WHO, Lyons, 2002.

Kimmonds *et al.,* 'Fruit and vegetable intake among adolescents and adults in the US: Percentage meeting individualized recommendations', *The Medscape Journal of Medicine*, 2009, vol. 11, page 26.

Lewis *et al.*, 'Predictors of depressed mood in spouses of women with breast cancer', *Journal of Clinical Oncology*, 2008, vol. 26, pages 1289-95.

National Research Council, *Diet and Health: Implications for Reducing Chronic Disease Risk*, 1989, http://www.nap.edu/catalog.php?record_id=1222, accessed 27 July 2010.

Reynolds *et al.*, 'Active smoking, household passive smoking and breast cancer: Evidence from the California Teachers Study', *Journal of the National Cancer Institute*, 2004, vol. 96, pages 29-37.

Royal College of Radiologists, *Interactions between cancer treatment and herbal and nutritional supplements and medicines: Information for doctors*, 2006, http://www.rcr.ac.uk/docs/oncology/pdf/herbalsupplementsfinalversion.pdf, accessed 27 July 2010.

Thorogood, M *et al.,* 'Risk of death from cancer and ischaemic heart disease in meat and non-meat eaters', *BMJ*,1994, vol. 308, pages 1667-70.

World Health Organisation (WHO), *Programmes and Projects: Cancer*, http://www.who.int/cancer/en/, accessed 14 Oct 2010.

Zang *et al.*, 'Alcohol Consumption and Breast Cancer Risk in the Women's Health Study', *American Journal of Epidemiology*, 2007, vol. 165, issue 6, pages 667-76.